# Palgrave Studies in Science and Popular Culture

Series editor
Sherry Vint
University of California, Riverside
Riverside, CA, USA

This book series seeks to publish ground-breaking research exploring the productive intersection of science and the cultural imagination. Science is at the centre of daily experience in twenty-first century life and this has defined moments of intense technological change, such as the Space Race of the 1950s and our very own era of synthetic biology. Conceived in dialogue with the field of Science and Technology Studies (STS), this series will carve out a larger place for the contribution of humanities to these fields. The practice of science is shaped by the cultural context in which it occurs and cultural differences are now key to understanding the ways that scientific practice is enmeshed in global issues of equity and social justice. We seek proposals dealing with any aspect of science in popular culture in any genre. We understand popular culture as both a textual and material practice, and thus welcome manuscripts dealing with representations of science in popular culture and those addressing the role of the cultural imagination in material encounters with science. How science is imagined and what meanings are attached to these imaginaries will be the major focus of this series. We encourage proposals from a wide range of historical and cultural perspectives.

**Advisory Board:**
Mark Bould, University of the West of England, UK
Lisa Cartwright, University of California, US
Oron Catts, University of Western Australia, Australia
Melinda Cooper, University of Sydney, Australia
Ursula Heise, University of California Los Angeles, US
David Kirby, University of Manchester, UK
Roger Luckhurt, Birkbeck College, University of London, UK
Colin Milburn, University of California, US
Susan Squier, Pennsylvania State University, US


More information about this series at
http://www.springer.com/series/15760

Evie Kendal · Basia Diug
Editors

# Teaching Medicine and Medical Ethics Using Popular Culture

palgrave
macmillan

*Editors*
Evie Kendal
Monash University
Melbourne, VIC, Australia

Basia Diug
Faculty of Medicine, Nursing and
   Health Sciences
Monash University
Melbourne, VIC, Australia

Palgrave Studies in Science and Popular Culture
ISBN 978-3-319-65450-8        ISBN 978-3-319-65451-5    (eBook)
DOI 10.1007/978-3-319-65451-5

Library of Congress Control Number: 2017949474

Cover credit: xmee

Printed on acid-free paper

This Palgrave Macmillan imprint is published by Springer Nature
The registered company is Springer International Publishing AG
The registered company address is: Gewerbestrasse 11, 6330 Cham, Switzerland

# Acknowledgements

The editors wish to thank all of the contributors for their insightful chapters and the Faculty of Medicine, Nursing and Health Sciences at Monash University for financially supporting this project through the Learning and Teaching Research Grant Scheme. Thanks are also due to the Monash Education Academy for providing support for the editors to present research from this project at the International Society for the Scholarship of Teaching and Learning (ISSoTL) Conference and the Council of Academic Public Health Institutions Australia (CAPHIA) Learning and Teaching Forum, and we acknowledge the invaluable feedback we received from peers at both of these events. We are also grateful to all the staff, students and industry professionals who gave their time to complete surveys and interviews for the various studies reported in this collection, without whom this research could not have been completed. Finally, we wish to acknowledge the valuable feedback received from the anonymous peer-reviewers for the collection.

# CONTENTS

1 Introduction: The Use of Popular Culture
in Medical and Health Education                                    1
Evie Kendal and Basia Diug

2 Hidden in Plain Sight: Family Presence During
Resuscitation on Prime-Time Media                                17
Zohar Lederman

3 The *ER* Effect: How Medical Television Creates
Knowledge for American Audiences                                 37
Jessica Bodoh-Creed

4 WhyZombie? Zombie Pop Culture to Improve
Infection Prevention and Control Practices                       55
Peta-Anne Zimmerman and Matt Mason

5 Celebrity? Doctor? Celebrity Doctor? Which
Spokesperson is Most Effective for Cancer Prevention?           71
Candice-Brooke Woods, Stacey Baxter, Elizabeth King,
Kerrin Palazzi, Christopher Oldmeadow and Erica L. James

6   An Empirical Study of Student Engagement with
    Professional and Ethical Issues in Medical Television
    Dramas                                                          99
    Evie Kendal and Basia Diug

7   Teaching Millennials: A Three-Year Review of the
    Use of Twitter in Undergraduate Health Education               115
    Basia Diug and Evie Kendal

8   Balancing the Needs of the Many Against the Needs
    of the Few: Aliens, Holograms and Discussions
    of Medical Ethics                                              133
    Allie Ford and Lynette Pretorius

9   Mind-Melds and Other Tricky Business: Teaching
    Threshold Concepts in Mental Health Preservice
    Training                                                       149
    Lynette Pretorius and Allie Ford

Index                                                              169

# EDITORS AND CONTRIBUTORS

## About the Editors

**Evie Kendal** is a feminist bioethicist and literary critic from Melbourne, Australia. She is currently a Lecturer at the School of Public Health and Preventive Medicine, Monash University, Alfred Centre, Melbourne, Australia, where she teaches into the Bachelor of Health Science and Bachelor of Biomedical Science degree programmes. Evie's research focuses on the representation of ectogenesis and other reproductive biotechnologies in popular culture and the impact this has on public policy and the bioethical debates surrounding these technologies. She is the author of *Equal Opportunity and the Case for State Sponsored Ectogenesis* (Palgrave Macmillan, 2015) and 'Utopian Visions of "Making People": Science Fiction and Debates on Cloning, Ectogenesis, Genetic Engineering, and Genetic Discrimination,' in *Biopolitics and Utopia: An Interdisciplinary Reader*, ed. Patricia Stapleton and Andrew Byers (Palgrave Macmillan, 2015).

**Basia Diug** is Senior Lecturer, School of Public Health and Preventive Medicine, Monash University, Alfred Centre, Melbourne, Australia, and Deputy Head of the Medical Education Research and Quality unit (MERQ). She joined the School of Public Health and Preventive Medicine in 2006. She has extensive experience in both quantitative and qualitative research methods, as well as research design and project management. She has a particular interest in medication safety through the identification of adverse events both at an individual and system level.

## Contributors

**Stacey Baxter** is Associate Professor of Marketing for the Newcastle Business School at the University of Newcastle, Australia. She holds a Ph.D. in Management (Marketing) from the University of Newcastle. Stacey has published in international academic journals such as the *International Journal of Research in Marketing, European Journal of Marketing, Journal of Advertising, Marketing Letters, International Journal of Market Research* and the *Journal of Consumer Marketing.*

**Jessica Bodoh-Creed** is a medical and media anthropologist who is currently a Lecturer in the Department of Anthropology at California State University, Los Angeles in the Department of Anthropology. Her research focuses on knowledge production within medical media from television to pharmaceutical advertising to celebrity physicians and promotion. She received her Ph.D. in Anthropology from the University of California, Riverside.

**Allie Ford** is a Learning Skills Adviser at Monash University, Australia. She works with academics to integrate academic skills development and training into the curriculum. She also teaches at both undergraduate and postgraduate levels in a range of academic disciplines, including Medicine, Nursing and Health Sciences. Allie has qualifications in Astrophysics, Chemistry and Education, and her research interests include the scholarship of teaching and learning, assessment, reflective practice, transition and curriculum design.

**Erica L. James** is an Associate Professor and Convenor of the Master of Public Health programme at University of Newcastle, Callahan, Australia. She teaches health promotion and interactional skills to both undergraduate and postgraduate students. Erica has qualifications in Exercise Science, Health Promotion and Behavioural Epidemiology, and her research focus is behavioural nutrition and physical activity in relation to cancer prevention and control.

**Elizabeth King** has broad experience across the public and not-for-profit health sectors. She has particular experience in policy development and programme evaluation in relation to population health and cancer prevention initiatives.

**Zohar Lederman** is a medical intern at Sourasky Medical Center, Tel Aviv, Israel, and a Ph.D. candidate at the National University of Singapore. His areas of interest include family presence during resuscitation, One Health, and ethics of public health and infectious diseases.

**Matt Mason** is a Lecturer at the School of Nursing, Midwifery & Paramedicine, University of the Sunshine Coast. Peta-Anne and Matt are both experienced, credentialled Infection Prevention and Control Professionals and Registered Nurses, in both acute and public health settings. Both have been trained and deployed overseas by the WHO Global Outbreak Alert and Response Network. Both are pop-culture geeks, and proud.

**Christopher Oldmeadow** is the Senior Statistician at the Hunter Medical Research Institute, New South Wales, Australia. He has a Bachelor degree in Mathematics/Statistics and a Ph.D. in Statistics. He provides statistical expertise for projects from various fields of medical research, ranging from basic science, through to health services research and preventative public health programmes.

**Kerrin Palazzi** is a statistician with the CReDITSS (Clinical Research Design, Information Technology and Statistical Support) group at Hunter Medical Research Institute, New South Wales, Australia. She works with researchers and students to provide statistical analysis and research methodology support; this has resulted in co-authorship of over 70 journal articles in a diverse range of topics including quality of life studies, behavioural interventions, nutritional studies, oncology outcomes, animal model studies, mental health and addiction research, and randomised clinical trials. Kerrin has qualifications in biomedical science and public health and her research interests include statistics, epidemiology, public health and cancer research.

**Lynette Pretorius** is the Academic Language Development Advisor for the Faculty of Education at Monash University, Australia. She works with both undergraduate and postgraduate students to improve their academic language proficiency and literacy skills. Lynette has qualifications in Medicine, Science, Education and Counselling, and her research interests include experiential learning, self-efficacy, doctoral education, curriculum design, heart failure and atrial fibrillation.

**Candice-Brooke Woods** is a Ph.D. candidate (Behavioural Science in Relation to Medicine) at the University of Newcastle. Candice has qualifications in Nursing and Marketing and her research interests include social marketing, spokesperson effects and behaviour change in relation to preventative cancer and non-profit advertising.

**Peta-Anne Zimmerman** is a Lecturer in the Graduate Infection Prevention and Control Programme, School of Nursing and Midwifery, Griffith University, Australia. She is also Visiting Research Fellow, Gold Coast Hospital and Health Service, and Member of Menzies Health Institute, Queensland, Australia. Peta-Anne holds a position on the Australasian College for Infection Prevention and Control (ACIPC) Credentialling and Professional Standards Committee. Peta-Anne and Matt are both experienced, credentialled Infection Prevention and Control Professionals and Registered Nurses, in both acute and public health settings. Both have been trained and deployed overseas by the WHO Global Outbreak Alert and Response Network. Both are pop-culture geeks, and proud.

# List of Figures

Fig. 4.1    Incidence of zombie films of infectious cause                                    59

Fig. 5.1    Example mock print PSA stimuli—medical doctor
            (study one) (*Mock print PSA stimuli for this study were
            created by adapting an original resource developed by the
            Cancer Council South Australia, and use of the Program
            name 'SunSmart' developed by the Cancer Council Victoria.
            Spokesperson images sourced from iStock by Getty Images.*)    77

Fig. 5.2    Example mock print PSA stimuli—medical doctor (study two)
            (*Mock print PSA stimuli for this study were created by adapting
            an original resource developed by the Cancer Council South
            Australia, and use of the Program name 'SunSmart' developed
            by the Cancer Council Victoria. Spokesperson images sourced
            from iStock by Getty Images.*)                               78

Fig. 5.3    Mediation analysis: Celebrity versus medical doctor (part one)    80

Fig. 5.4    Mediation analysis: Celebrity doctor versus medical doctor
            (part two)                                                   81

Fig. 6.1    Student television watching behaviours by show:
            *Grey's Anatomy, House, M.D.* and *Scrubs*                   105

Fig. 6.2    Student television watching behaviours by method/source      105

Fig. 6.3    Student television viewing behaviours                        106

Fig. 6.4    Positive and negative representations of certain
            professional qualities and behaviours                       108

Fig. 7.1    Reported use of social media platforms prior to the study    120

Fig. 7.2    Comparison of prior use of social media and other
            online tools for BMS students in 2016                       121

Fig. 7.3    Students' perception of staff accessibility and
            Twitter-related assessment (Likert scales where strongly
            agree = 1, agree = 2, disagree = 3 and strongly
            disagree = 4)                                                    123
Fig. 7.4    Students' perception of peer collaboration and
            Twitter-related assessment (Likert scales where strongly
            agree = 1, agree = 2, disagree = 3, and strongly
            disagree = 4)                                                    124

# LIST OF TABLES

Table 2.1   Characteristics of CPR cases                                     21
Table 5.1   Health spokesperson effects (part one): Summary
            of crude means (SD)                                              79
Table 5.2   Mediating effects of health spokesperson expertise
            and familiarity on behavioural intention (part one)             80
Table 5.3   Participant spokesperson preference (count % within
            participant group) (part one)                                   81
Table 5.4   Health spokesperson effects (part one): Summary
            of crude means (SD)                                             82
Table 5.5   Mediating effects of health spokesperson expertise
            and familiarity on behavioural intention (part two)             83
Table 5.6   Participant spokesperson preference (count % within
            participant group) (part two)                                   83
Table 6.1   Student demographic characteristics by degree                  103
Table 6.2   Student television watching and behaviours by degree           104
Table 6.3   Students' perceptions on accuracy and how appropriately
            issues are handled in medical television programmes             107
Table 6.4   Perceived influence of medical television shows on
            forming opinions                                               109
Table 7.1   Cohort demographic characteristics across the
            three-year period 2014–2016                                    120
Table 7.2   Student self-report thoughts on appropriateness
            and engagement across the three years                          122
Table 7.3   Percentage of students' perception of staff accessibility      123
Table 7.4   Percentage of students' perception of peer collaboration       124

## CHAPTER 1

# Introduction: The Use of Popular Culture in Medical and Health Education

*Evie Kendal and Basia Diug*

There is an increasing awareness of the role of mass media and popular culture in communicating health information to the general public and medical students.[1] Medical television series in particular have been identified as a rich source of health information and medical ethics training, depicting doctor–patient relationships that are both entertaining and educational. Recent research has shown that these fictional representations of the medical profession have an impact on perceptions of real-life doctors, and can influence recruitment of students into medical, nursing and health science degrees.[2] Beginning with CBS's *City Hospital* in 1951, medical television dramas have remained a staple of prime-time television.[3] In his book, *Medicinema*, Brian Glasser notes that popular film culture and medicine have always been intricately connected, with film historians placing the first representations of medical personnel in fictional films before that of 'cowboys, criminals or the clergy.'[4] With such a historically entrenched relationship between fact and fiction, it is unsurprising that medical dramas regularly come under scrutiny regarding their potential influence on public perceptions of doctors and the

E. Kendal (✉) · B. Diug
Monash University, Melbourne, VIC, Australia
e-mail: evie.kendal@monash.edu

© The Author(s) 2017
E. Kendal and B. Diug (eds.), *Teaching Medicine and Medical Ethics Using Popular Culture*, Palgrave Studies in Science and Popular Culture, DOI 10.1007/978-3-319-65451-5_1

health system.[5] Furthermore, there is ongoing debate regarding the usefulness of televised medicine in medical and health science curriculum, with Roslyn Weaver and Ian Wilson reporting that university educators often seem concerned about 'how the fictional world of medicine intrudes on and influences the real one.'[6]

The purpose of this edited collection is to discuss the use of popular culture in medical education, paying particular attention to medical television dramas. While there are many aspects of popular culture that go beyond television, Victoria Rideout notes that:

> As a communications tool, TV continues to dominate, primarily because the size of its audience is unrivaled, dwarfing that of even the most popular websites. But hard evidence about the impact of so-called "edu-tainment" is hard to come by, and opportunities for large-scale, nationally representative evaluations of health messages in TV shows are rare.[7]

These difficulties are present both when evaluating the impact of popular television on the general public, as well as for medical and health students. With many tertiary education providers moving towards more evidence-based pedagogical practices, there is an urgent need to explore how educators are engaging with popular culture and the impact this is having on students' learning. This process has been under way for some time, with previous studies demonstrating various methods of incorporating popular culture into university teaching and health communication more generally. The studies contained within this collection add to this knowledge base, in addition to providing practical teaching tips for educators in this field looking to exploit the power of popular media, while simultaneously avoiding some of the pitfalls associated with it. As such, it would be beneficial to first briefly review the results of recent research on this topic. This introduction will then conclude with a summary of each of the chapters in the collection.

## How has Popular Culture been Used in Medical Education?

At its most basic, 'popular culture' can be defined as the cultural and artistic expressions that appeal to a large audience, whose dissemination is often facilitated through mass media, and which is generally distinguished somehow from 'high' or 'elite' culture.[8] The most common use of popular culture reported in the medical education literature involves using episodes of popular medical television dramas in the place of more traditional case studies. Pablo Blasco et al. claim this method generates classroom discussion in a similar way to problem-based learning activities.[9] These discussions also occur outside the classroom, when students and members of the general public engage with these shows and talk about the medical and ethical issues portrayed in them. As such, Weaver et al. claim that medical television forms part of the 'informal curriculum' of medicine, exposing students to new perspectives about how medicine can or should be practised.[10] With a particular focus on medical ethics training, Angelo Volandes notes:

> Film offers a powerful and underutilised medium in which clinical vignettes come alive in their rich and textured details, both medical and non-medical … Phrases often appearing in written vignettes, such as "aggressive procedures" and "futile care", lose their amorphous qualities as students see and experience ventilators and medical emergencies on the screen.[11]

Other authors agree that television episodes may be better suited to generating discussion than the short written scenarios often used in medical education. Jeffery Spike claims that this only works if the audience sees the whole story, rather than just a short clip, as familiarity with the television characters is essential for teasing out the complexities of the issues they face as doctors and patients.[12] He relates how an episode of *Scrubs* ('My Fifteen Seconds') was inspired by contemporary studies that showed doctors typically interrupted their patients after just 12–18 seconds, even though most patients would be able to convey their full message within 26–30 seconds if allowed to speak uninhibited.[13] The consequences of such an affront to the model doctor–patient relationship are conveyed well in the episode, in part because the series' lead doctor, J.D., is the one who must come to the realisation that he was wrong when he said an average of fifteen seconds per patient was 'all the time you need.' When he almost loses a patient because he didn't take the time to hear her whole story, he finally learns that as a doctor 'you can never underestimate the importance of listening'—a lesson the viewer learns alongside him.[14] As the lovable, but flawed, fictional doctor, J.D. personifies the real-life doctors in those studies on average listening times, showing viewers not only how these situations come to be common in medical practice, but also why we should be campaigning to change them. Such a poignant message is likely to stay with all viewers, but particularly those embarking on the very career depicted in the show. However, for the episode to have its full effect it must be watched in its entirety.

If devoting a significant proportion of an already limited class time to watching or discussing a medical television series, it is necessary to first have clear learning objectives in mind. Similarly, if hoping to use popular culture references to communicate health information to the lay public, evidence of the efficacy of this technique is needed. Two examples in the literature stand out as particularly well designed in this matter: one focused on teaching non-clinician epidemiologists about medical issues, and the other on educating the general public on HIV transmission rates. The first was a study by Truls Østbye et al. in 1997, in which epidemiologists and biostatisticians were asked to watch episodes of *ER* in tutorials. As stated by the authors, the established goals of this educational intervention were 'to illustrate referral bias and other epidemiological issues in a clinical setting' and 'to provide human faces to the disease data students usually work with.'[15] As it was deemed impractical for these students to attend ward rounds, the fictional clinical setting of *ER* was used as a substitute, with students expected to record presenting symptoms and demographic information on the patients admitted in the episodes. The results of the study indicated students found the sessions interesting and informative, and that they provided a useful comparison between what diseases are most prevalent in the real world, versus those which get the most screen time in popular media, with a disproportionate number of trauma cases admitted as opposed to patients with chronic illnesses.[16] A similar trend has been observed in news media coverage of health conditions and medical research, with the more dramatic and rare injuries and diseases being reported on with greater frequency, a trend that has been shown to affect public perceptions of disease risk.[17]

The second example noted above is more recent, and involved surveying *Grey's Anatomy* viewers to ascertain the educational impact of an episode focused on maternal-fetal HIV transmission rates. This study was completed by the Kaiser Family Foundation in 2008, and clearly demonstrated the educational potential of medical television dramas for a general audience.[18] First, members of the Foundation with expertise in HIV and pregnancy briefed the show's writers, who then incorporated the issue of maternal-fetal HIV transmission into an episode ('Piece of

My Heart') that first aired on 1 May, 2008. The episode follows Izzie, one of the series' regular doctors, as she cares for an HIV-positive patient who has just discovered she is pregnant. Believing her child will inevitably be infected by the virus, the patient requests an abortion. Izzie then makes numerous attempts to communicate to the patient that the real risk of transmission is very low if she is taking her standard medications throughout the pregnancy. Eventually Izzie convinces the patient it is safe for her to proceed with the pregnancy, stating: 'I wasn't saying there's *some* chance your baby might not be sick. I'm saying there is a 98% chance your baby will be born perfectly healthy. *Ninety-eight percent.*'[19] Before the episode aired only 15% of survey respondents asked to estimate the likelihood of a healthy baby being born in this situation selected 'more than a 90% chance.' One week after viewing the episode this rose to 61%, with 45% still selecting this option six weeks after the episode.[20] Attitudes toward HIV-positive pregnant women were also investigated, with 61% of respondents before the episode stating it was irresponsible for an HIV-positive woman to have a baby, a figure which dropped to 34% the week after the episode aired. Survey items that were on the same topic but which were not directly referenced in the episode showed no change over the six-week period.[21]

Looking beyond television, celebrity and social media are also sources of health information for students and the general public. There has long been awareness that celebrities have the capacity to reach vast audiences with their health messages, representing an opportunity for effective health promotion, but also bringing fears regarding accuracy and safety.[22] Angelina Jolie's highly publicised prophylactic double mastectomy in 2013, for example, encouraged many women to seek testing for the BRCA1 and BRCA2 gene mutations associated with increased risk of breast cancer, with one hereditary cancer clinic in New South Wales, Australia, recording a 300–400% increase in referrals for the six weeks following Jolie's announcement.[23] This figure remained elevated a year later, with a 200% increase on the numbers of referrals compared to previous years. This became known as the 'Angelina Effect,' and inspired the Cancer Council Victoria to deliver an informative webinar regarding the true proportion of breast cancer cases in Australia linked to genetic factors (5–10%).[24] Despite the potential to exaggerate concerns regarding the BRCA mutations, Jolie's advocacy increased awareness of a real health risk; however, there have also been a number of celebrity health campaigns that both students and the general public may have been exposed to in recent memory, which were based on fraudulent or dangerous claims. One example includes that of 'wellness' blogger, Belle Gibson, who deceived a mass online following into believing she had cured her terminal cancer through holistic medicine and healthy eating. Gibson made a fortune from her 'The Whole Pantry' app and cookbook, which Consumers Affairs Victoria alleged was made through 'false and misleading representations,' and she has also been accused of failing to deliver charitable donations from her followers.[25] What is most interesting about both of these examples is how mass media communication facilitated the dissemination of health information, but not the necessary education to critically appraise the accuracy or relevance of this information to the audience. This highlights an opportunity within the health education sector to provide such analytical skills for students, as future health practitioners and educators themselves.

While the dominant focus of this collection is the use of popular television dramas, owing to their pervasive presence in medical curricula, contemporary celebrity health stories and scandals make interesting case studies to discuss in the classroom. There will also be some discussion of the role of social media, such as Twitter, on increasing health awareness among students and the general public, owing to the extensive reach such media have. This will intersect with recent developments in gamification for health promotion, including through gaming apps such as Metro Trains Victoria's 'Dumb Ways to Die,' a rail safety promotion mobile game.

## WHY IS POPULAR CULTURE USED IN MEDICAL EDUCATION?

Doctors exist in popular culture as symbols of the chaotic influence of disease and death on people's lives, both within the fictional world and in reality. Sickness often features in drama to heighten the emotions of the viewer as they identify with suffering patients and their families.[26] But why do fictional doctors and illnesses appear in medical education? For Østbye et al. *ER* was used for convenience as it provided a means of communicating medical information to methodologists that didn't require hospital placements.[27] They note that prior to the 1950s such an intervention would not have been necessary, as the majority of epidemiologists were already physicians who just happened to engage in simple quantitative studies on the side. However, as epidemiological methods increased in sophistication the two fields diverged, meaning those trained in advanced quantitative methods often required greater collaboration with biologists and clinicians to conduct their research.[28] Their study was intended to bridge some of this knowledge gap and provide a common language for such collaborations.

Another benefit of using popular television in the classroom is its capacity to evoke emotion and sympathy in viewers, qualities patients often accuse their doctors of lacking. Blasco et al. claim there is 'growing concern that the human dimension of the physician is receding in the face of ever-emerging technological advances,' noting that when patients report being dissatisfied with their care this often 'points more to the human deficiencies of medical professionals than to their technical shortcomings.'[29] Using as a pedagogical tool a medium that many medical and health students already regularly engage with, captures their interest and emotions in a way lectures and case studies are unlikely to manage.[30] Anna Pavlov and Gregory Dahlquist also note that unlike the isolated classroom case study, the 'continuity of the television series' allows students to follow the lives of fictional doctors and patients over an extended period of time, providing a parallel to the practice of family medicine.[31] Surveys on medical students conducted by Weaver et al. also demonstrate that students are exposed to many issues related to professionalism and ethics through medical television series, and that they may draw from these fictional experiences when forming their identity as physicians.[32] They note that:

> With careful selection, medical television dramas can engage students with important professionalism issues which are usually too abstract in the formal curriculum but perhaps too threatening in the clinical environment.[33]

It is important to remember that medical, nursing and health science students learn from their exposure to medical television, whether or not there is any deliberate attempt to include it in university curricula. The conscious use of popular culture in the classroom provides a valuable opportunity to mediate between students and the knowledge they receive from such media. Michael O'Connor further claims that series such as *ER* might provide pre-clinical students with 'their most vivid glimpse into the practice of medicine,' noting that a medical student who regularly watches the show over their four year medical degree will spend as much time engaged in this activity as in emergency medicine rotations.[34] Importantly, students might be exposed to clinical and ethical issues in fictional media that may never arise during their limited hospital placements, providing an opportunity to discuss these issues as students before having to face them in practice.[35]

## WHAT IS THE EFFECT OF USING POPULAR CULTURE IN MEDICAL EDUCATION?

While previous research on the subject suggests many medical students are unaware of any influence of popular culture on their medical education, the high levels of consumption and recall within this cohort seem to indicate they are retaining information learned from these sources.[36] This has caused concern among some medical educators who question the accuracy of these shows. In 2009, two clinicians wrote a letter to the editor of the journal *Resuscitation* citing concerns about the frequency of suboptimal positioning of patients for endotracheal intubation. When surveying student doctors regarding their training in the area, the authors found that 'after "trial and error", a surprising number answered that television medical dramas had been an important influence,' with *ER* being the most common source.[37] On analysing 22 instances of the technique in the show, the authors determined that 'none (0/22) achieved more than one, let alone all three, components of optimal airway positioning.'[38] The potential for real-world impact is alarming, and indicates medical teaching facilities should be addressing what happens in these shows to prevent misinformation from negatively impacting patient care. Other authors relate that unrealistic expectations of the efficacy of cardio-pulmonary resuscitation, for doctors and patients alike, might stem in part from the frequency with which fictional patients survive after CPR. In an article for the *Journal of the American Medical Association* in 1998, O'Connor considered various studies in which long-term survival rates following CPR in television programmes including *ER*, *Chicago Hope* and *Rescue 911* were as high as 67%; meanwhile actual survival rates reported in the medical literature at the time were less than 15%.[39] The glamourisation of emergency medicine in these shows has also been implicated in changing recruitment patterns across specialities, especially since the premiere of *ER* in 1994.[40]

With regard to the impact of popular culture on the dissemination of health information for the general public, the Kaiser Family Foundation's study of *Grey's Anatomy* is again a useful example to consider. Of the regular viewers surveyed, 45% reported learning something new about a health issue from watching the show and 17% of all viewers said they had sought further information on a topic they'd seen depicted, many seeking out health professionals to discuss the issue.[41] Rideout notes that since episodes of *Grey's Anatomy* average 20 million viewers, more than three million may have pursued a health issue on the basis of this exposure.[42] Extrapolating from the 46% increase in awareness of maternal-fetal HIV transmission rates seen in the first week following the target episode yields a total of over eight million people potentially educated on this issue by the show.[43] It is hard to imagine most medical journal articles having anywhere near this degree of influence. It also suggests that current and future doctors need to be made aware of the impact of popular culture on their patients' level of knowledge regarding certain health conditions.

Regarding popular television more generally, in 2005 the Centers for Disease Control and Prevention (CDC) released an Executive Summary of the Porter Novelli HealthStyles survey investigating the impact of popular television programmes on health education in the general population (n = 3479), with 67% of regular daytime drama viewers and 58% of regular prime-time drama viewers reporting learning something new about a health issue or disease from a television show in the previous six months. A further 8% of respondents reported learning about a health issue or disease from another person describing a television episode to them.[44] The report concludes that television dramas and comedies are powerful educational tools, and that the format of these shows promotes personal identification with the characters in a way that 'enhances learning and prevention' through 'parasocial interaction.'[45] As such, professionals responsible for educating the general public on health matters might benefit from the opportunity to understand how popular culture functions as an educational tool beyond the traditional classroom setting.

According to Katherine Foss, public perceptions of the medical profession have also followed trends in popular media. She refers to studies claiming that from the 1950s to the 1970s fictional doctors were typically portrayed as heroes, with heavy viewers of medical dramas reporting higher levels of trust for health professionals than people who either didn't watch these shows or who did so only occasionally.[46] She claims that as these representations have changed in news and popular media, so have attitudes and beliefs about health professionals in the real world. She particularly draws attention to the potential influence of medical television series on underestimations of the rate of medical errors occurring in medical practice, and beliefs regarding the reasons behind such errors when they do arise.[47] Other studies have also shown that medical dramas can influence organ donation rates and the time taken before seeking emergency medical attention for conditions such as chest pain.[48]

## Chapter Summaries

This collection opens with a chapter by Zohar Lederman, which focuses on the potential impact of representations of cardio-pulmonary resuscitation (CPR) in popular television on healthcare providers' perceptions toward whether family members should be present during this procedure. Comparing the official guidelines to depictions in medical television dramas, Lederman traces a shift in how family presence during CPR has been represented over time. In the second chapter, Jessica Bodoh-Creed notes how the 'CSI Effect' has been linked to jury members' inflated expectations of the role of forensic evidence in criminal trials, and argues for a similar impact on patients' expectations through what she terms the '*ER* Effect.' The third chapter continues this theoretical approach to the role of popular culture in medical education, with Peta-Anne Zimmerman and Matt Mason evaluating the representation of infection prevention and control measures in zombie narratives. Candice-Brooke Woods et al. then consider the potential risks and benefits of using celebrity spokespeople rather than medical doctors in cancer prevention campaigns and social marketing. Across these chapters there is a critical focus on the impact of popular culture broadly conceived to include film, television, social media and celebrity culture.

The second half of this collection is focused on providing further practical examples for how educators can use popular culture in the classroom, beginning with two chapters by the collection's editors. The first looks at the potential to use medical television dramas for tertiary education, based on an analysis of the level of consumption and awareness of ethical and medical issues arising in these programs among health, biomedical and medical students. The second addresses how social media engagements and mobile gaming apps can be effectively embedded into formal curricula, to provide future health practitioners the skills they need to engage with this form of health promotion. The collection closes with two chapters by Allie Ford and Lynette Pretorius, focused on how to use *Star Trek* to teach foundational medical ethics, and threshold concepts for patient-centred care in the mental health care sector. As a long-running film and television franchise incorporating both completed and continuing series, *Star Trek* is widely known and thus accessible to many audiences. The medical television dramas included throughout this section are likewise a mix of completed and ongoing series, satisfying different requirements for narrative closure and currency.

## NOTES

1. Roslyn Weaver, Ian Wilson and Vicki Langendyk, 'Medical Professionalism on Television: Student Perceptions and Pedagogical Implications,' *Health* 18, no. 6 (2014): 600.
2. Ibid., 609; Roslyn Weaver and Ian Wilson, 'Australian Medical Students' Perceptions of Professionalism and Ethics in Medical Television Programs,' *BMC Medical Education* 11 (2011): 50; Matthew J. Czarny, Ruth R. Faden and Jeremy Sugarman, 'Bioethics and Professionalism in Popular Television Medical Dramas,' *Journal of Medical Ethics* 36 (2010): 203.
3. Tae Kyoung Lee and Laramie D. Taylor, 'The Motives For and Consequences of Viewing Television Medical Dramas,' *Health Communication* 29 (2014): 13; Tim Brooks and Earle Marsh, *The Complete Directory to Prime Time Network and Cable TV Shows 1946–Present* (New York: Ballantine Books, 2007), 257.
4. Brian Glasser, *Medicinema: Doctors in Films* (Oxford: Radcliffe Publishing, 2010), 1.
5. Anna Pavlov and Gregory E. Dahlquist, 'Teaching Communication and Professionalism Using a Popular Medical Drama,' *Family Medicine* 42, no. 1 (2010): 25.
6. Weaver and Wilson, 'Australian Medical Students,' 54.
7. Victoria Rideout, 'Television as a Health Educator: A Case Study of Grey's Anatomy,' A Kaiser Family Foundation Report, September 2008, 1.
8. A variety of definitions are outlined and evaluated in Dominic Strinati's *An Introduction to Theories of Popular Culture*, 2nd edition (London and New York: Routledge, 1995).
9. Pablo G. Blasco, Cauê F. Mônaco, Maria Auxiliadora C. De Benedetto, Graziela Moreto and Marcelo R. Levites, 'Teaching Through Movies in a Multicultural Scenario: Overcoming Cultural Barriers Through Emotions and Reflection,' *Family Medicine* 42, no. 1 (2010): 24.
10. Weaver, Wilson and Langendyk, 'Medical Professionalism,' 607.

11. Angelo Volandes, 'Medical Ethics on Film: Towards a Reconstruction of the Teaching of Healthcare Professionals,' *Journal of Medical Ethics* 33 (2007): 678–9.
12. Jeffery Spike, 'Television Viewing Habits and Ethical Reasoning: Why Watching *Scrubs* Does a Better Job than Most Bioethics Classes,' *The American Journal of Bioethics* 8, no. 12 (2008): 11–12.
13. *Ibid.*, 11.
14. *Scrubs*, 'My Fifteen Seconds,' Episode 7, Season 3. Directed by Ken Wittingham. Written by Mark Stegeman. NBC, 20 November 2003.
15. Truls Østbye, Bill Miller and Heather Keller, 'Throw that Epidemiologist out of the Emergency Room! Using the Television Series *ER* as a Vehicle for Teaching Methodologists about Medical Issues,' *Journal of Clinical Epidemiology* 50, no. 10 (1997): 1184.
16. Ibid., 1185.
17. Meredith E. Young, Geoffrey R. Norman and Karin R. Humphreys, 'Medicine in the Popular Press: The Influence of the Media on Perceptions of Disease,' *PLoS ONE* 3, no. 10, e3552. doi: 10.1371/journal.pone.0003552; David F. Ransohoff and Richard M. Ransohoff, 'Sensationalism in the Media: When Scientists and Journalists May be Complicit Collaborators,' *Effective Clinical Practice* 4, no. 4 (2001): 185.
18. Rideout, 'Television as a Health Educator,' 2.
19. *Grey's Anatomy*, 'Piece of My Heart,' Episode 13, Season 4. Directed by Mark Tinker. Written by Stacy McKee. ABC, 1 May 2008.
20. Rideout, 'Television as a Health Educator,' 3.
21. Ibid., 6.
22. Judith A. Baker, Cyndi J. Lepley, Satya Krishnan and Kathryn S. Victory, 'Celebrities as Health Educators: Media Advocacy Guidelines,' *Journal of School Health* 62, no. 9 (1992): 433.
23. Kate Dunlop, Judy Kirk and Kathy Tucker, 'In the Wake of Angelina – Managing a Family History of Breast Cancer,' *Australian Family Physician* 43, nos. 1–2 (2014): 76.
24. Ibid.; Cancer Council Victoria, 'Angelina Jolie and genetic breast cancer risk,' 15 May 2013, available at: http://www.cancervic.org.au/about/media-releases/2013-media-releases/may-2013/angelina-jolie.html.
25. Karen Percy, 'Belle Gibson May have been Delusional when Blogging Fake Brain Cancer Claims: Court,' *ABC News*, 15 March 2017, available at: http://www.abc.net.au/news/2017-03-15/belle-gibson-wellness-blogger-decision-handed-down/8355236.
26. Glasser, *Medicinema*, 122.
27. Østbye et al. 'Throw that Epidemiologist,' 1183–4.
28. Ibid., 1183.
29. Blasco et al. 'Teaching Through Movies,' 22.

30. Weaver, Wilson and Langendyk, 'Medical Professionalism,' 599.
31. Pavlov and Dahlquist, 'Teaching Communication,' 25.
32. Weaver, Wilson and Langendyk, 'Medical Professionalism,' 608; Weaver and Wilson, 'Australian Medical Students,' 50.
33. Ibid.
34. Michael M. O'Connor, 'The Role of the Television Drama *ER* in Medical Student Life: Entertainment or Socialization?' *JAMA* 280, no. 9 (1998): 854.
35. Matthew J. Czarny, Ruth R. Faden, Marie T. Nolan, Edwin Bodensiek and Jeremy Sugarman, 'Medical and Nursing Students' Television Viewing Habits: Potential Implications for Bioethics,' *American Journal of Bioethics* 8, no. 12 (2008): 7.
36. Weaver and Wilson, 'Australian Medical Students,' 53–4.
37. P.G. Brindley and C. Needham, 'Positioning Prior to Endotracheal Intubation on a Television Medical Drama: Perhaps Life Mimics Art,' [letter to the editor] *Resuscitation* 80 (2009): 604.
38. Ibid.
39. O'Connor, 'The Role of the Television Drama,' 854.
40. Ibid.
41. Rideout, 'Television as a Health Educator,' 5–6.
42. Ibid., 9.
43. Ibid., 8.
44. Centers for Disease Control and Prevention, 'TV Drama/Comedy Viewers and Health Information 2005 Porter Novelli Healthstyles Survey: Executive Summary,' *HealthStyles* (2005): 1–2.
45. Ibid., 3.
46. Katherine A. Foss, '"When we make mistakes, people die!": Constructions of Responsibility for Medical Errors in Televised Medical Dramas, 1994–2007,' *Communication Quarterly* 59, no. 4 (2011): 487.
47. Ibid., 502.
48. Bruce B. Dan, 'TV or not TV: Communicating Health Information to the Public,' [editorial] *JAMA* 268, no. 8 (1992): 1027.

## BIBLIOGRAPHY

Baker, Judith A., Cyndi J. Lepley, Satya Krishnan and Kathryn S. Victory. 'Celebrities as Health Educators: Media Advocacy Guidelines.' *Journal of School Health* 62, no. 9 (1992): e433.
Blasco Pablo G., Cauê F. Mônaco, Maria Auxiliadora C. De Benedetto, Graziela Moreto and Marcelo R. Levites. 'Teaching Through Movies in a Multicultural Scenario: Overcoming Cultural Barriers Through Emotions and Reflection.' *Family Medicine* 42, no. 1 (2010): 22–4.

Brindley, P.G. and C. Needham. 'Positioning Prior to Endotracheal Intubation on a Television Medical Drama: Perhaps Life Mimics Art.' [letter to the editor] *Resuscitation* 80 (2009): 604.

Brooks, Tim and Earle Marsh. *The Complete Directory to Prime Time Network and Cable TV Shows 1946–Present.* New York: Ballantine Books, 2007.

Cancer Council Victoria. 'Angelina Jolie and genetic breast cancer risk.' (15 May 2013), available at: http://www.cancervic.org.au/about/media-releases/2013-media-releases/may-2013/angelina-jolie.html.

Centers for Disease Control and Prevention. 'TV Drama/Comedy Viewers and Health Information 2005 Porter Novelli Healthstyles Survey: Executive Summary.' *HealthStyles*, 2005.

Czarny, Matthew J., Ruth R. Faden and Jeremy Sugarman. 'Bioethics and Professionalism in Popular Television Medical Dramas.' *Journal of Medical Ethics* 36 (2010): 203–6.

Czarny, Matthew J., Ruth R. Faden, Marie T. Nolan, Edwin Bodensiek and Jeremy Sugarman. 'Medical and Nursing Students' Television Viewing Habits: Potential Implications for Bioethics.' *American Journal of Bioethics* 8, no. 12 (2008): 1–8.

Dan, Bruce B. 'TV or not TV: Communicating Health Information to the Public.' [editorial] *JAMA* 268, no. 8 (1992): 1026–7.

Dunlop, Kate, Judy Kirk and Kathy Tucker. 'In the Wake of Angelina – Managing a Family History of Breast Cancer.' *Australian Family Physician* 43, nos. 1–2 (2014): 76–8.

Foss, Katherine A. '"When we make mistakes, people die!": Constructions of Responsibility for Medical Errors in Televised Medical Dramas, 1994–2007.' *Communication Quarterly* 59, no. 4 (2011): 484–506.

Glasser, Brian. *Medicinema: Doctors in Films.* Oxford: Radcliffe Publishing, 2010.

*Grey's Anatomy*, 'Piece of My Heart,' Episode 13, Season 4. Directed by Mark Tinker. Written by Stacy McKee. ABC, 1 May 2008.

Lee, Tae Kyoung and Laramie D. Taylor. 'The Motives For and Consequences of Viewing Television Medical Dramas.' *Health Communication* 29 (2014): 13–22.

O'Connor, Michael M. 'The Role of the Television Drama *ER* in Medical Student Life: Entertainment or Socialization?' *JAMA* 280, no. 9 (1998): 854–5.

Østbye, Truls, Bill Miller and Heather Keller. 'Throw that Epidemiologist out of the Emergency Room! Using the Television Series *ER* as a Vehicle for Teaching Methodologists about Medical Issues.' *Journal of Clinical Epidemiology* 50, no. 10 (1997): 1183–6.

Pavlov, Anna and Gregory E. Dahlquist. 'Teaching Communication and Professionalism Using a Popular Medical Drama.' *Family Medicine* 42, no. 1 (2010): 25–7.

Percy, Karen. 'Belle Gibson May have been Delusional when Blogging Fake Brain Cancer Claims: Court.' *ABC News*, 15 March 2017, available at: http://www.abc.net.au/news/2017-03-15/belle-gibson-wellness-blogger-decision-handed-down/8355236.

Ransohoff David F. and Richard M. Ransohoff. 'Sensationalism in the Media: When Scientists and Journalists May be Complicit Collaborators.' *Effective Clinical Practice* 4, no. 4 (2001): 185–8.

Rideout, Victoria. 'Television as a Health Educator: A Case Study of Grey's Anatomy.' A Kaiser Family Foundation Report, September 2008.

*Scrubs*, 'My Fifteen Seconds,' Episode 7, Season 3. Directed by Ken Wittingham. Written by Mark Stegeman. NBC, 20 November 2003.

Spike, Jeffery. 'Television Viewing Habits and Ethical Reasoning: Why Watching *Scrubs* Does a Better Job than Most Bioethics Classes.' *The American Journal of Bioethics* 8, no. 12 (2008): 11–13.

Strinati, Dominic. *An Introduction to Theories of Popular Culture*, 2nd edition. London and New York: Routledge, 1995.

Volandes, Angelo. 'Medical Ethics on Film: Towards a Reconstruction of the Teaching of Healthcare Professionals.' *Journal of Medical Ethics* 33 (2007): 678–80.

Weaver, Roslyn and Ian Wilson. 'Australian Medical Students' Perceptions of Professionalism and Ethics in Medical Television Programs.' *BMC Medical Education* 11 (2011): 50–5.

Weaver, Roslyn, Ian Wilson and Vicki Langendyk. 'Medical Professionalism on Television: Student Perceptions and Pedagogical Implications.' *Health* 18, no. 6 (2014): 597–612.

Young, Meredith E., Geoffrey R. Norman and Karin R. Humphreys. 'Medicine in the Popular Press: The Influence of the Media on Perceptions of Disease.' *PLoS ONE* 3, no. 10, e3552. doi: 10.1371/journal.pone.0003552.

## CHAPTER 2

# Hidden in Plain Sight: Family Presence During Resuscitation on Prime-Time Media

*Zohar Lederman*

The first episode of the third season of *Heroes* begins when Peter Petrelli is excluded from the hospital room where his brother, Nathan Petrelli, is undergoing cardiopulmonary resuscitation (CPR).[1] The doctor who escorts him out does not even reply to the question, 'is he going to make it?' and closes the doors to the room without a word. The background music expresses urgency. In the next scene, Peter watches helplessly as the disappointed doctor comes out of the room and utters, 'I'm sorry.'

Family presence during cardiopulmonary resuscitation remains a much contested topic in clinical ethics. Even though professional guidelines support it, healthcare professionals commonly oppose it and decline to implement the guidelines. The reasons for this opposition include the perception that CPR is chaotic, bloody, and that relatives might become obstructive and/or faint. Interestingly, the author's personal experience suggests that even students of the medical professions or medical professionals who have minimal or no experience with CPR share this negative

Z. Lederman (✉)
National University of Singapore,
Singapore, and Sourasky Medical Center, Tel Aviv, Israel
e-mail: zoharlederman@gmail.com

© The Author(s) 2017
E. Kendal and B. Diug (eds.), *Teaching Medicine and Medical Ethics Using Popular Culture*, Palgrave Studies in Science and Popular Culture, DOI 10.1007/978-3-319-65451-5_2

attitude towards family presence during CPR. This chapter explores the origins of this attitude. Specifically, it empirically examines one plausible origin for the predominant negative attitude among students of the health professions or junior medical professionals towards family presence during CPR—prime-time media.

For the purpose of this chapter, the following definitions will be used:

- CPR in the media: Any situation in which chest compressions or emergency intubation were performed on a patient; a patient was said to be having 'an arrest' or be 'crashing'; an unconscious patient was treated for a life-threatening arrhythmia; or a physician declares a patient dead.
- FPDR (Family Presence During Resuscitation): The ability of any family member (blood related or not), friend, spouse or anyone who shares some form of intimate relationship with the patient to watch, talk and/or touch the patient.

Importantly, this chapter focuses on adult CPR, excluding paediatric CPR from the discussion. While the differences between the two populations are not necessarily morally significant, most studies implicitly distinguish the two.[2] Therefore, to prevent any potential biases and circumvent potential objections, only adult CPR will be discussed.

## FAMILY PRESENCE DURING RESUSCITATION

Guidelines recommending parameters for allowing families to be present during adult CPR were published in the USA as early as 1994.[3-5] Currently, both European and American nursing and medical guidelines recommend allowing FPDR.[6-10] A recent report by the Institute of Medicine also advocates for FPDR.[11] Two recent large studies demonstrated the lack of negative effects of FPDR on in-hospital CPR outcome and the benefits FPDR holds for relatives.[12-14] However, FPDR is still not widely endorsed by healthcare professionals around the world.[15] In fact, in 2003 only 5% of 984 American nurses who participated in a survey worked in critical care/emergency units that had protocols allowing FPDR.[16] The literature suggests that while the majority of nurses oppose FPDR, they favour it more than physicians. Further, less experienced physicians are less likely to favour FPDR.[17-24]

Healthcare providers commonly raise a variety of reasons against FPDR, including: concern for the family experiencing a traumatic event;

concern for the privacy and care of patients; increased law suits against healthcare staff; lack of physical space at the bedside; or concern for professional staff that might experience performance anxiety or be subjected to acts of violence by relatives.[20,25-27]

While empirical evidence and ethical deliberation have debunked the majority of these concerns, this chapter will not attempt to engage with them directly.[28] Rather, the questions that concern us here are the following: How do healthcare professionals form these (mis)conceptions? Particularly, the author's personal experience suggests that medical students, who never participated in CPRs, tend to instinctively oppose FPDR. But whence do they learn this 'intuition'? This chapter does not presume to answer these questions completely, but rather seeks to discuss one medium, which may create and fuel oft-misguided perceptions of and attitudes towards FPDR. In short, I suggest in this chapter that television may influence the attitudes of laypeople as well as medical professionals and students towards FPDR.

## MEDICAL DRAMAS AND MEDICAL SOCIALISATION

Medical dramas have long been considered a major vector of medical information which shape and contribute to the social appearance and cultural influence of the medical institution.[29] As early as 1996, Diem et al. suggested that the false portrayal of CPR on television instils upon the public an unrealistic notion of its success rates and hence gives a false sense of hope.[30] Other observational studies that examined different television shows, both American and foreign, have demonstrated that the success rates of CPR were in fact realistic but suggested other concerns, such as: the psychological qualitative (rather than quantitative) effects of dramatic CPR scenes,[31] unrealistic reasons for CPR and type of population undergoing resuscitation,[32,33] and failure to depict long-term effects rather than short term ones.[34] Specifically, laypersons' perceptions of FPDR and CPR in general might also be affected by television, as might be inferred from Grice et al.[35]

Moreover, many have discussed the specific effects that medical dramas have on medical students, such as causing more students to choose a specific residency,[36] or shaping their medical conduct in general.[37] One study calls to change the way in which the healthcare system is depicted in medical dramas, for fear that viewers might have false expectations from their healthcare providers.[38] Another study congratulates the scriptwriters of *House, M.D.* for their realistic depiction of chronic-pain management.[39] Even Baer, a physician and co-producer of *ER*, who, in reply to Diem et al. warned against blaming television rather than the physicians themselves, still affirms that television affects viewers' knowledge, at least to some extent.[40]

## STUDY DESCRIPTION

I sought to analyse how FPDR is depicted in prime-time medical dramas, the reasoning being that these dramas often provide students of medical professions with their first encounter with CPR. For this purpose, I watched and analysed the first season of *House, M.D.* (22 episodes),[41] and *Grey's Anatomy* (nine episodes).[42] For comparison, I also analysed 16 episodes of *Medic*. *Medic* was the first hit prime-time medical drama aired in the USA, between 1954 and 1956, while *House* (2004–2012) and *Grey's Anatomy* (2005–present) are among the most popular prime-time medical dramas to date.[29] I identified CPR cases according to the definition stated above and for each case recorded seven items: name, age and sex of patient, cause of CPR, underlying illness, location of CPR and details of family presence. A second academic observer reviewed five episodes of *House, M.D.* in order to increase internal validity. I reviewed the results a second time to further increase internal validity. CPRs in the operating room (OR) were excluded, on the assumption that family could not be present under those circumstances.

The results were as follows (see Table 2.1):

*House: M.D*: 14 CPRs were recorded, of which one was performed in a pre-hospital setting. In four of the CPRs there is no family at the bedside. In one of these cases, the family member (business agent) appears right after intubation and complains that it was done despite a do not resuscitate (DNR) order. In four cases family members are excluded, either by escorting them out of the room or by shutting the blinds. In six cases family members are present, one of which occurred in a pre-hospital setting. In one case out of these six cases, relatives (nuns) are not present in the room but allowed to watch from the outside with open blinds. Family members are never invited to be present during CPR. In none of the six cases where family is present are they accompanied by a member of the staff.

*Grey's Anatomy*: 12 CPRs were recorded (two CPRs which took place in the OR were not considered). In ten cases there are no family members at the bedside during CPR. In one case the family member (wife) is

**Table 2.1**  Characteristics of CPR cases

| CPR | Episode | Name | Age | Sex | Cause | Underlying illness at the time of CPR | Location | Details of family presence |
| --- | --- | --- | --- | --- | --- | --- | --- | --- |
| House 1 | Pilot | Rebecca Adler | Young adult | F | Seizure | Unknown | Hospital | None |
| House 2 | 'Occam's razor' | Brandon | 16 | M | Ventricular tachycardia during heart catheterisation | Unknown | Hospital clean room | Parents are watching from outside and seem confused/frightened after the physician shuts the blinds |
| House 3 | 'Maternity' | Hartig | Neonate | F | Seizure | Unknown | Hospital | Parents are present and are not excluded |
| House 4 | 'Maternity' | Chen-Lupino | Neonate | F | Infection | Unknown | Hospital clean room | Family member waits outside and blinds get shut |
| House 5 | 'Damned if you do' | Sister Augustine | Adult | F | Tachycardia | Unknown | Hospital | Other nuns are present and House does not exclude them |
| House 6 | 'Damned if you do' | Sister Augustine | Adult | F | Anaphylactic reaction | Unknown | Hospital clean room | Other nuns watch from outside |

(continued)

**Table 2.1** (continued)

| CPR | Episode | Name | Age | Sex | Cause | Underlying illness at the time of CPR | Location | Details of family presence |
|---|---|---|---|---|---|---|---|---|
| House 7 | 'Poison' | Matt | Adolescent | M | Bradycardia | Unknown | Hospital | Mother is in the room, asked to move aside by the physician but is not excluded |
| House 8 | 'Poison' | Chi | Adolescent | M | Unknown | Unknown | Hospital | Parents are escorted out |
| House 9 | 'DNR' | John Henry | Old | M | Iatrogenic | ALS? | Hospital | Agent comes in after intubation and resents CPR despite of 'DNR' order |
| House 10 | 'Cursed' | Gabe Reilich | 12 | M | Laryngospasm | Anthrax? | Hospital | Parents are in the room, father doubts the physicians while the mother calms him down ('Let them do their job') |

(continued)

**Table 2.1** (continued)

| CPR | Episode | Name | Age | Sex | Cause | Underlying illness at the time of CPR | Location | Details of family presence |
|---|---|---|---|---|---|---|---|---|
| House 11 | 'Control' | Carly | Young | F | Respiratory arrest during angiography | Unknown | Hospital | None |
| House 12 | 'Heavy' | Jessica | 10 | F | Myocardial infarction | Unknown | School | Other students are present |
| House 13 | 'Babies and bath water' | Naomi | Young adult | F | Pulmonary embolism | Small cell carcinoma | Hospital | Husband is escorted out |
| House 14 | 'Three stories' | Unknown | Middle age | M | Allergic reaction to antivenom | Snake bite | Hospital | None |
| *Medic* 1 | 'General practitioner' | Unknown | Old | M | Unknown | Strokes | Home | Rabbi and daughter are present |
| Grey's 1 | 'A hard day's night' | Katie Bryce | Young adult | F | Seizure | Epilepsy | Hospital | None |
| Grey's 2 | 'The first cut is the deepest' | Allison | Young adult | F | Rape | Unknown | Hospital | None |
| Grey's 3 | 'The first cut is the deepest' | Unknown | 57 | M | Asystole | Unknown | Hospital | None |
| Grey's 4 | 'The first cut is the deepest' | Unknown | Unknown | ? | Unknown | Unknown | Hospital | None |
| Grey's 5 | 'The first cut is the deepest' | Unknown | Unknown | ? | Unknown | Unknown | Hospital | None |

(continued)

**Table 2.1** (continued)

| CPR | Episode | Name | Age | Sex | Cause | Underlying illness at the time of CPR | Location | Details of family presence |
|---|---|---|---|---|---|---|---|---|
| Grey's 6 | 'Winning a battle, losing the war' | Kevin Davidson | Middle age | M | Trauma | Bike race | Hospital | Wife comes in while patient is in a coma after CPR |
| Grey's 7 | 'No man's land' | Liz | 55 | F | Pancreatic cancer | Pancreatic cancer | Hospital | None |
| Grey's 8 | 'Shake your groove on' | Mrs. Patterson | Old | F | Post-coronary artery bypass graft | Unknown | Hospital | Husband is asked to leave by the physician ('Get him out of here') but does not |
| Grey's 9 | 'If tomorrow never comes' | Jimmie Harper | Late middle age | M | Thrombo-embolism | Post-chest tube placement | Hospital | Wife is present during the collapse but is escorted out during CPR |
| Grey's 10 | 'The self destruct button' | 'Digby' Owens | Young adult | M | Septic shock | A tattoo | Hospital | None |
| Grey's 11 | 'Save me' | Unknown | Young | F | Unknown | Unknown | Hospital | None |
| Grey's 12 | 'Who's zoomin' who' | Mr. Franklin | Old | M | Complication of paracentesis | Hepatic failure | Hospital | None |

present, but is escorted out of the room. In one case, the family member is asked by the physician to leave the room, but does not comply. Family is never invited to be present during CPR. In the one case in which one family member is present (husband), there is no staff member to accompany him.

*Medic*: One CPR was recorded, in which the physician comes to the patient's home and declares him dead, with no intervention. The patient's daughter is sitting at the bedside; a rabbi is present as well.

## DISCUSSION

Two conclusions can be drawn from the results. The first is that current prime-time medical dramas do not portray the option of FPDR as recommended by current guidelines. However, these medical dramas are realistic insofar as they present a negative stance towards FPDR, which is the prevailing medical practice worldwide.[16–22] In both dramas, no family members were ever invited to be present during CPR. On *Grey's Anatomy*, in one case family members were asked to leave the room during CPR. In all other ten cases of CPR no family members were present. FPDR is only allowed in one out of 12 CPRs, and only because of the family member's insistence. In *House*, family members were present in six out of 14 CPRs, and were not present in four other cases. In four cases the family was excluded. In those five in-hospital CPRs where family was present in the room or allowed to watch from outside, there was no staff member to support them, as recommended by professional guidelines.[6,7] As mentioned earlier, in one case the family member (business agent) enters the room after an emergency intubation is performed on a patient who signed a DNR order. The agent is clearly (and rightly) upset.

A second conclusion, albeit anecdotal at most owing to low statistical power ($n = 1$), is that CPR in *Medic* is portrayed in a very different manner than it is in *House* and *Grey's Anatomy*.[43–46] The patient lies in his bed, in his home, with his daughter and a rabbi who prays while the patient is dying. Once he dies, the physician does not attempt any heroic measures, but simply covers the patient's face with a blanket and turns immediately to console the daughter, affirming that they have discussed the issue before and that it was 'bound to happen.'[47] The grieving process of the family begins in the same room where death was announced, and at the same time, together with the body of the loved one, the physician and a supporting figure (in this case, a rabbi). The background music is quiet and soothing, unlike the hectic music that appears in most of the CPRs that occur in the more modern shows (this, of course, could not have been quantified objectively).

Drawing from these two conclusions, one may assume the effects these modern medical dramas might have on patients, their families and medical professionals, especially those with less real-life experience, such as medical students and interns. Family members are rarely present, and if they are present they are escorted out of the room in a dramatic manner: music is hectic, blinds are shut and the stressed physician uses an assertive tone and strong language, for example exclaiming 'Get him out of here!' The DNR case in *House* further emphasises this point: the family member realises that the physician disobeyed the law (as well as ignored the patient's autonomy) and is therefore legally liable. The viewer might conclude that family members are either almost never present at the bedside or that they are (and ought to be) excluded from their loved one's CPR by escorting them out of the room and/or by shutting the blinds. Moreover, the viewer might wrongly deduce that FPDR would increase the risk of a legal lawsuit and that family members might lose their calm and interfere with the patient's care (see Gabe Reilich case in *House*, where the father publicly and vocally doubts and threatens the physicians).[12,48,49]

Of course, the aforementioned is far from proving a causative effect. Similar to the argument presented by Baer,[40] there is no evidence that the way FPDR is depicted in prime-time television actually affects either the public's or healthcare professionals' attitudes towards the issue, so no real causal correlation can be established at the moment.

Two more general points should be noted. First, 16 episodes of *Medic* depict only one case of CPR, while the current medical dramas depict many more. Second, in *Medic* the dying takes place at home and no intervention is made by the physician, while in the current medical dramas dying usually happens inside the hospital and rigorous CPR is performed. As many have suggested, it seems reasonable to assume that this modern over-medicalisation of death and dying originates both from advancements in technology and, to a larger extent, a change in the modern cultural notion of death and medicine's role in coping with it.[50] Modern society has become afraid of death (subconsciously or consciously), and instead of facing this fear it turns to the comforting image of the hospital and the white coat. In the hospital, death can take place behind the curtain, meaning out of sight. Relatives often bring their loved ones to the hospital with no clear expectations or, worse yet, with false expectations as to treatment options and prognosis. Furthermore, relatives often believe that by taking their loved ones to the hospital they will have maximised the patient's well-being.[46,51–55] Sadly, this is far from true.[56,57]

What are we then to do? From a descriptive perspective, medical dramas seem to portray the status quo realistically: relatives are commonly excluded from their loved one's CPR. From a normative perspective, however, medical dramas fail to portray what *should* be the status quo based on empirical evidence, professional guidelines and ethical deliberation.[28] Potentially, this may create, or perpetuate, misconceptions about the effects of FPDR among medical professionals as well as among laypeople.

Do the non-medical personnel responsible for these medical dramas— that is, the producers, screenwriters and so on—have a moral obligation to portray FPDR according to empirical data and professional guidelines? I believe so, but my intention is not to argue for it here. Rather, this chapter is mainly addressed to medical professionals or students who are either involved in the production of these shows or who are watching these shows. I join with Baer,[40] and Diem et al.[30] by arguing that physicians and other healthcare professionals bear a great responsibility in countering the inaccurate images portrayed on television and should educate patients, their families and themselves about the risks (or lack thereof) and benefits of FPDR. This responsibility is threefold. First, those healthcare professionals who consult with screenwriters should push toward a more accurate depiction of FPDR. Second, healthcare professionals ought to offer the option of FPDR and verify that family members are well informed and know what to expect, regardless of their decision. Third, healthcare professionals should educate their colleagues, particularly the less experienced ones, about the benefits of FPDR and refer them to current guidelines.

## Conclusion

Patients and less experienced healthcare professionals have few sources from which to learn about FPDR. Even though a causal correlation between FPDR on television and its effects on FPDR in real life has not been established, it is likely to be an influencing factor. The study described here suggests that medical dramas, while realistic in this sense, do not portray FPDR as they should, in a way that is beneficial to both staff members and families. Screenwriters should be aware of this, and perhaps consider modifying the manner in which they portray FPDR. More importantly, medical professionals should educate themselves and their colleagues about the benefits of FPDR and apply professional guidelines to their practice. Medical professionals who advise screenwriters should push for a depiction of FPDR that is more congruent with existing empirical evidence—misconceptions help no one.

After discussing an *ER* scene in which Dr Kerry Weaver dramatically excludes a patient's mother from the resuscitation of her son, Ellen Tsai argues that:

> Art imitates life. Our traditional practice during resuscitation procedures is to exclude family members, keeping them out of the room until we have ceased our efforts. Why do physicians and nurses continue to deny family member the option of staying with patients while they are dying, even though the results of numerous studies favor the family's presence? It is time for us to stop hiding behind unfounded fears.[58]

I concur, and I would add that occasionally it is life that imitates art.

## NOTES

1. *Heroes*, 'The Second Coming,' Episode, 1, Season 3. Directed by Allan Arkush. Written by Tim Kring. NBC, 22 September 2008.
2. Reasons for this distinction fall beyond the scope of this article.
3. R.O. Cummins and M.F. Hazinski, 'The Most Important Changes in the International ECC and CPR Guidelines 2000,' *Circulation* 102 (2000): 371–6.
4. American Heart Association, 'ECC Guidelines Part 2: Ethical Aspects of CPR and ECC,' *Circulation* 102 (2000): 12–21.
5. Emergency Nurses Association, 'Position Statement: Family Presence at the Bedside During Invasive Procedures and Cardiopulmonary Resuscitation' (1994), available at: https://www.ena.org/SiteCollectionDocuments/Position%20Statements/Archived/FamilyPresence.pdf.
6. P. Fulbrook, J. Latour, J. Albarran, W. de Graaf, F. Lynch, D. Devictor et al. 'The Presence of Family Members During Cardiopulmonary Resuscitation: European federation of Critical Care Nursing Association, European Society of Paediatric and Neonatal Intensive Care and

European Society of Cardiology Council on Cardiovascular Nursing and Allied Professions Joint Statement,' *EJCN* 6 (2007): 255–8.

7. L.J. Morrison, G. Kierzek, D.S. Diekema, M.R. Sayre, S.M. Silvers, A.H. Idris et al. 'Part 3: Ethics: 2010 American Heart Association Guidelines for Cardiopulmonary Resuscitation and Emergency Cardiovascular Care,' *Circulation* 122 (2010): 665–75.

8. Resuscitation Council, UK, *Should Relatives Witness Resuscitation? A report from a Project Team of the Resuscitation Council (UK)*, London: Resuscitation Council, UK (1996), available at: https://www.resus.org.uk/archive/archived-cpr-information/should-relatives-witness-resuscitation/.

9. L.L. Bossaert, G.D. Perkins, H. Askitopoulou, V.I. Raffay, R. Greif, K.L. Haywood et al. 'European Resuscitation Council Guidelines for Resuscitation 2015: Sect. 11. The Ethics of Resuscitation and End-of-life decisions,' *Resuscitation*, 95 (2015): 302–11.

10. The recently published 2015 guidelines by the American Heart Association (AHA), while still supporting FPDR, use a language that is far weaker than AHA guidelines from previous years: 'Overall, given the evidence for improved psychological benefits for families present during out-of-hospital resuscitation, and without an apparent negative effect on outcomes at hospitals that allow families to be present, family presence represents an important dimension in the paradigm of resuscitation quality': M.E. Kleinman, E.E. Brennan, Z.D. Goldberger, R.A. Swor, M. Terry, B.J. Bobrow et al. 'American Heart Association Guidelines for Cardiopulmonary Resuscitation and Emergency Cardiovascular Care: Adult Basic Life Support and Cardiopulmonary Resuscitation Quality,' *Circulation* 132 (2015): s424.

11. R. Graham, M.A. McCoy, A.M. Schultz, eds. *Strategies to Improve Cardiac Arrest Survival: A Time to Act* (Washington: National Institutes of Health, 2015).

12. P. Jabre, V. Belpomme, E. Azoulay, L. Jacob, L. Bertrand, F. Lapostolle et al. 'Family Presence during Cardiopulmonary Resuscitation,' *New Engl. J. Med.* 368, no. 11 (2013): 1008–18.

13. P. Jabre, K. Tazarourte, S.W. Borron, V. Belpomme, L. Jacob, L. Bertrand et al. 'Offering the Opportunity for Family to be Present During Cardiopulmonary Resuscitation: 1-Year Assessment,' *Intensive Care Med.* 40 (2014): 981–7.

14. Z.D. Goldberger, B.K. Nallamothu, G. Nichol, P.S. Chan, J.R. Curtis and C.R. Cooke, 'Policies Allowing Family Presence During Resuscitation and Patterns of Care During In-Hospital Cardiac Arrest,' *Circ. Cardiovasc. Qual. Outcomes* 8 (2015): 226–34.

15. J.A. Colbert and J.N. Adler, 'Family Presence during Cardiopulmonary Resuscitation—Polling Results,' *New Engl. J. Med.* 368, no. 26 (2013): e38.
16. S.L. MacLean, C.E. Guzzetta, C. White, D. Fontaine, T. Meyers and P. Desy, 'Family Presence During Cardiopulmonary Resuscitation and Invasive Procedures: Practices of Critical Care and Emergency Nurses,' *American Journal of Critical Care* 12 (2003): 246–57.
17. C.R. Duran, K.S. Oman, J.J. Abel, V.M. Koziel and D. Szymanski, 'Attitudes Toward and Beliefs about Family Presence: A Survey of Healthcare Providers, Patients' Families, and Patients,' *American Journal of Critical Care* 16 (2007): 270–9.
18. A. Badir and D. Sepit, 'Family Presence during CPR: A Study of the Experiences and Opinions of Turkish Critical Care Nurses,' *Int. J. Nurs. Stud.* 44 (2010): 83–92.
19. O. Wacht, K. Dopelt, Y. Snir and N. Davidovitch, 'Attitudes of Emergency Department Staff toward Family Presence during Resuscitation,' *I.M.A.J.*, 12, no. 6 (2010): 366–70.
20. M.A. Halm, 'Family Presence During Resuscitation: A Critical Review of the Literature,' *American Journal of Critical Care* 14 (2005): 494–511.
21. C.K. Sheng, C.K. Kim and A. Rashidi, 'A Multi-center Study on the Attitudes of Malaysian Emergency Health Care Staff Towards Allowing Family Presence during Resuscitation of Adult Patients,' *Int. J. Emerg. Med.* 3 (2010): 287–91.
22. B.M. McClenathan, K.G. Torrington, and C.F.T. Uyehara, 'Family Member Presence during Cardiopulmonary Resuscitation: A Survey of US and International Critical Care Professionals,' *Chest* 122 (2002): 2204–211.
23. C.D. Critchell and P.E. Marik, 'Should Family Members Be Present During Cardiopulmonary Resuscitation? A Review of the Literature,' *Am. J. Hosp. Palliat. Care* 24, no. 4 (2007): 311–17.
24. Z. Manzar and M. Siddique, 'Presence of Family Members During Cardio-Pulmonary Resuscitation after Necessary Amendments,' *J. Pak. Med. Assoc.* 58 (2008): 632–5.
25. O. Wacht, 'The Attitudes of the Emergency Department Staff Toward Family Presence During Resuscitation,' M.H.A, Health Systems Management (Beer-Sheva: Ben-Gurion University of the Negev, 2008).
26. J. Boehm, 'Family Presence During Resuscitation,' *Code Communications* 3, no. 5 (2008).
27. Z. Lederman and O. Wacht, 'Family Presence During Resuscitation: Attitudes of Yale-New Haven Hospital Staff,' *Yale J. Biol. Med.* 87, no. 1 (2014): 63–72.

28. Z. Lederman, M. Garasic and M. Piperberg, 'Family Presence During Cardiopulmonary Resuscitation: Who Should Decide?,' *J. Med. Ethics* 40 (2014): 315–19.

29. See, for example: J. Turow, *Playing Doctor: Television, Storytelling, & Medical Power*, 2nd edn (Michigan: The University of Michigan Press, 2010).

30. S.J. Diem, J.D. Lantos and J.A. Tulsky, 'Cardiopulmonary Resuscitation on Television: Miracles and Misinformation,' *New Engl. J. Med.* 334 (1996): 1578–82.

31. J. Van Den Bulck and K. Damiaans, 'Cardiopulmonary Resuscitation on Flemish Television: Challenges to the Television Effects Hypothesis,' *Emerg. Med. J.* 21, no. 5 (2004): 565–7.

32. P.N. Gordon, S. Williamson and P.G. Lawler, 'As Seen on TV: Observational Study of Cardiopulmonary Resuscitation in British Television Medical Drama,' *B.M.J.* 317 (1998): 780–3.

33. R.J. Market and M.G. Saklayen, 'Correspondence—Cardiopulmonary Resuscitation on Television,' *New Engl. J. Med.* 335, no. 21 (1996): 1605–13.

34. D. Harris and H. Willoughby, 'Resuscitation on Television: Realistic or Ridiculous? A Quantitative Observational Analysis of the Portrayal of Cardiopulmonary Resuscitation in Television Medical Drama,' *Resuscitation* 80 (2009): 1275–9.

35. A.S. Grice, P. Picton and C.D.S. Deakin, 'Study Examining Attitude of Staff, Patients and Relatives to Witnessed Resuscitation in Adult Intensive Care Units,' *Br. J. Anaesth.* 91, no. 6 (2003): 820–4.

36. E.M. Wallack and G.J. Bingle, 'Correspondence—Cardiopulmonary Resuscitation on Television,' *New Engl. J. Med.* 335, no. 21 (1996): 1605–13.

37. M.M. O'Connor, 'The Role of the Television Drama ER in Medical Student Life: Entertainment or Socialization,' *J.A.M.A.* 280, no. 9 (1998): 854–5.

38. J. Turow, 'Television Entertainment and the US Health-care Debate,' *Lancet* 347 (1996): 1240–3.

39. J. Theivendran, *House M.D: An Analysis of Chronic Pain Managed with Opiate Therapy in Entertainment Television* (London: Imperial College Medical School, 2007).

40. N.A. Baer, ed. 'Cardiopulmonary Resuscitation on Television: Exaggerations and Accusations (editorial),' *New Engl. J. Med.* 334 (1996): 1604–6.

41. *House, M.D.* Season 1. Created by David Shore. Fox, 16 November 2004–24 May 2005.

42. *Grey's Anatomy*. Season 1. Created by Shonda Rhimes. ABC, 27 March 2005–22 May 2005.

43. Two important qualifications are worth nothing here. First, while appreciating the advantages of CPR as portrayed in *Medic*, it is imperative to note that chest compressions were only developed in the 1960s and mouth-to-mouth ventilation was still not standard of care. However, other CPR methods were being used.

44. S. Timmermans, *Sudden Death and the Myth of CPR*, 1st edn (Philadelphia, PA: Temple University Press, 1999).

45. International Guidelines 2000 Conference on Cardiopulmonary Resuscitation (CPR) and Emergency Cardiovascular Care (ECC), 'Introduction to the International Guidelines 2000 for CPR and ECC: A Consensus of Science,' *Circulation* 102 (2000): 1–11.

46. A.T. Nibert, 'Teaching Clinical Ethics Using a Case Study: Family Presence During Cardiopulmonary Resuscitation,' *Critical Care Nurse* 25 (2005): 38–44.

47. *Medic*. Created by James E. Moser. NBC, 13 September 1954–27 August 1956.

48. Again, it is imperative to note that none of these fears of FPDR has been substantiated in the literature.

49. C. Hanson and D. Strawser, 'Family Presence During Cardiopulmonary Resuscitation: Foote Hospital Emergency Department Nine-Year Perspective,' *Journal of Emergency Nursing* 18 (1992): 104–6.

50. There are cultural exceptions to this trend but it is a dominant shift.

51. H.M. Spiro, M.G. McCrea Curnen and L.P. Wandel, eds. *Facing Death: Where Culture, Religion and Medicine Meet* (New Haven, CT: Yale University Press, 1996).

52. E. Kübler-Ross, *On Death and Dying: What the Dying Have to Teach Doctors, Nurses, Clergy, and Their Own Families* (New York: Scribner, 2003).

53. S. Nuland, *How We Die: Reflections on Life's Final Chapter*, 2nd edn (New York: A.A. Knopf, 1994).

54. S. Timmermans, 'Resuscitation Technology in The Emergency Department: Towards a Dignified Death,' *Sociol. Health Illn.* 20, no. 2 (1998): 144–67.

55. S. Gupta, *Cheating Death: The Doctors and Medical Miracles that Are Saving Lives Against All Odds* (New York: Grand Central Life & Style, 2009).

56. A.F. Connors Jr, N.V. Dawson, N.A. Desbiens, W.J. Fulkerson Jr, L. Goldman, W.A. Knaus et al. 'A Controlled Trial to Improve Care for Seriously Ill Hospitalized Patients: The Study to Understand Prognoses

and Preferences for Outcomes and Risks of Treatments (SUPPORT),' *J.A.M.A.* 274, no. 20 (1995): 1591–8.

57. S.A. Khan, B. Gomes and I.J. Higginson, 'End-of-Life Care- What Do Cancer Patients Want?,' *Nat. Rev. Clin. Oncol.* 11 (2014): 100–8.
58. E. Tsai, 'Should Family Members Be Present During Cardiopulmonary Resuscitation?,' *New Engl. J. Med.* 346, no. 13 (2002): 1019–21.

**Acknowledgements** I would like to thank Jessica Hanser for assistance with the study and the writing of this manuscript.

## BIBLIOGRAPHY

American Heart Association. 'ECC Guidelines Part 2: Ethical Aspects of CPR and ECC.' *Circulation* 102 (2000): 12–21.

Badir, A. and D. Sepit. 'Family Presence During CPR: A Study of the Experiences and Opinions of Turkish Critical Care Nurses.' *International Journal of Nursing Studies* 44 (2010): 83–92.

Baer, N.A. 'Cardiopulmonary Resuscitation on Television: Exaggerations and Accusations (editorial).' *New England Journal of Medicine* 334 (1996): 1604–6.

Boehm, J. 'Family Presence During Resuscitation.' *Code Communications* 3, no. 5 (2008).

Bossaert, L.L., G.D. Perkins, H. Askitopoulou, V.I. Raffay, R. Greif, K.L. Haywood et al. 'European Resuscitation Council Guidelines for Resuscitation 2015: Section 11. The Ethics of Resuscitation and End-of-life decisions.' *Resuscitation* 95 (2015): 302–11.

Colbert, J.A. and J.N. Adler. 'Family Presence During Cardiopulmonary Resuscitation—Polling Results,' *New England Journal of Medicine* 368, no. 26 (2013): e38.

Connors Jr, A.F., N.V. Dawson, N.A. Desbiens, W.J. Fulkerson Jr, L. Goldman, W.A. Knaus et al. 'A Controlled Trial to Improve Care for Seriously Ill Hospitalized Patients: The Study to Understand Prognoses and Preferences for Outcomes and Risks of Treatments (SUPPORT).' *Journal of the American Medical Association* 274, no. 20 (1995): 1591–8.

Critchell, C.D. and P.E. Marik. 'Should Family Members Be Present During Cardiopulmonary Resuscitation? A Review of the Literature.' *American Journal of Hospice Palliative Care* 24, no. 4 (2007): 311–17.

Cummins, R.O. and M.F. Hazinski. 'The Most Important Changes in the International ECC and CPR Guidelines 2000.' *Circulation* 102 (2000): 371–6.

Diem, S.J., J.D. Lantos and J.A. Tulsky. 'Cardiopulmonary Resuscitation on Television: Miracles and Misinformation.' *New England Journal of Medicine* 334 (1996): 1578–82.

Duran, C.R., K.S. Oman, J.J. Abel, V.M. Koziel and D. Szymanski. 'Attitudes Toward and Beliefs about Family Presence: A Survey of Healthcare Providers, Patients' Families, and Patients.' *American Journal of Critical Care* 16 (2007): 270–9.

Emergency Nurses Association. 'Position Statement: Family Presence at the Bedside During Invasive Procedures and Cardiopulmonary Resuscitation' (1994), available at: https://www.ena.org/SiteCollectionDocuments/Position%20Statements/Archived/FamilyPresence.pdf.

Fulbrook, P., J. Latour, J. Albarran, W. de Graaf, F. Lynch, D. Devictor et al. 'The Presence of Family Members During Cardiopulmonary Resuscitation: European federation of Critical Care Nursing Association, European Society of Paediatric and Neonatal Intensive Care and European Society of Cardiology Council on Cardiovascular Nursing and Allied Professions Joint Statement.' *European Journal of Cardiovascular Nursing* 6 (2007): 255–8.

Goldberger, Z.D., B.K. Nallamothu, G. Nichol, P.S. Chan, J.R. Curtis and C.R. Cooke. 'Policies Allowing Family Presence During Resuscitation and Patterns of Care During In-Hospital Cardiac Arrest.' *Circulation Cardiovascular Quality Outcomes* 8 (2015): 226–34.

Gordon, P.N., S. Williamson and P.G. Lawler. 'As Seen on TV: Observational Study of Cardiopulmonary Resuscitation in British Television Medical Drama.' *British Medical Journal* 317 (1998): 780–3.

Graham, R., M.A. McCoy and A.M. Schultz, eds. *Strategies to Improve Cardiac Arrest Survival: A Time to Act.* Washington: National Institutes of Health, 2015.

Grice, A.S., P. Picton and C.D.S. Deakin. 'Study Examining Attitude of Staff, Patients and Relatives to Witnessed Resuscitation in Adult Intensive Care Units.' *British Journal of Anaesthesia* 91, no. 6 (2003): 820–4.

Gupta, S. *Cheating Death: The Doctors and Medical Miracles that Are Saving Lives Against All Odds.* New York: Grand Central Life & Style, 2009.

Halm, M.A. 'Family Presence During Resuscitation: A Critical Review of the Literature.' *American Journal of Critical Care* 14 (2005): 494–511.

Hanson, C. and D. Strawser. 'Family Presence During Cardiopulmonary Resuscitation: Foote Hospital Emergency Department Nine-Year Perspective.' *Journal of Emergency Nursing* 18 (1992): 104–6.

Harris D. and H. Willoughby. 'Resuscitation on Television: Realistic or Ridiculous? A Quantitative Observational Analysis of the Portrayal of Cardiopulmonary Resuscitation in Television Medical Drama.' *Resuscitation* 80 (2009): 1275–9.

International Guidelines 2000 Conference on Cardiopulmonary Resuscitation (CPR) and Emergency Cardiovascular Care (ECC). 'Introduction to the International Guidelines 2000 for CPR and ECC: A Consensus of Science.' *Circulation* 102 (2000): 1–11.

Jabre, P., V. Belpomme, E. Azoulay, L. Jacob, L. Bertrand, F. Lapostolle et al. 'Family Presence During Cardiopulmonary Resuscitation.' *New England Journal of Medicine* 368, no. 11(2013): 1008–18.

Jabre, P., K. Tazarourte, S.W. Borron, V. Belpomme, L. Jacob, L. Bertrand et al. 'Offering the Opportunity for Family to be Present During Cardiopulmonary Resuscitation: 1-Year Assessment.' *Intensive Care Medicine* 40 (2014): 981–7.

Khan, S.A., B. Gomes and I.J. Higginson. 'End-of-Life Care- What Do Cancer Patients Want?,' *Nature Reviews Clinical Oncology* 11 (2014): 100–8.

Kleinman, M.E., E.E. Brennan, Z.D. Goldberger, R.A. Swor, M. Terry, B.J. Bobrow et al. 'American Heart Association Guidelines for Cardiopulmonary Resuscitation and Emergency Cardiovascular Care: Adult Basic Life Support and Cardiopulmonary Resuscitation Quality.' *Circulation* 132 (2015): s424.

Kübler-Ross, E. *On Death and Dying: What the Dying Have to Teach Doctors, Nurses, Clergy, and Their Own Families.* New York: Scribner, 2003.

Lederman, Z., M. Garasic and M. Piperberg. 'Family Presence During Cardiopulmonary Resuscitation: Who Should Decide?' *Journal of Medical Ethics* 40 (2014): 315–19.

Lederman, Z. and O. Wacht. 'Family Presence During Resuscitation: Attitudes of Yale-New Haven Hospital Staff.' *Yale Journal of Biology and Medicine* 87, no. 1 (2014): 63–72.

MacLean, S.L., C.E. Guzzetta, C. White, D. Fontaine, T. Meyers and P. Desy. 'Family Presence During Cardiopulmonary Resuscitation and Invasive Procedures: Practices of Critical Care and Emergency Nurses.' *American Journal of Critical Care* 12 (2003): 246–57.

Manzar, Z. and M. Siddique. 'Presence of Family Members During Cardio-Pulmonary Resuscitation after Necessary Amendments.' *Journal of Pakistan Medical Association* 58 (2008): 632–5.

Market, R.J. and M.G. Saklayen. 'Correspondence—Cardiopulmonary Resuscitation on Television.' *New England Journal of Medicine* 335, no. 21 (1996): 1605–13.

McClenathan, B.M., K.G. Torrington and C.F.T. Uyehara. 'Family Member Presence During Cardiopulmonary Resuscitation: A Survey of US and International Critical Care Professionals.' *Chest* 122 (2002): 2204–11.

Morrison, L.J., G. Kierzek, D.S. Diekema, M.R. Sayre, S.M. Silvers, A.H. Idris et al. 'Part 3: Ethics: 2010 American Heart Association Guidelines for Cardiopulmonary Resuscitation and Emergency Cardiovascular Care,' *Circulation* 122 (2010): 665–75.

Nibert, A.T. 'Teaching Clinical Ethics Using a Case Study: Family Presence During Cardiopulmonary Resuscitation.' *Critical Care Nurse* 25 (2005): 38–44.

Nuland, S. *How We Die: Reflections on Life's Final Chapter*, 2nd edn. New York: A.A. Knopf, 1994.

O'Connor, M.M. 'The Role of the Television Drama ER in Medical Student Life: Entertainment or Socialization.' *Journal of the American Medical Association* 280, no. 9 (1998): 854–5.

Resuscitation Council, UK. *Should Relatives Witness Resuscitation? A report from a Project Team of the Resuscitation Council (UK)* (1996), available at: https://www.resus.org.uk/archive/archived-cpr-information/should-relatives-witness-resuscitation/.

Sheng, C.K., C.K. Kim and A. Rashidi. 'A Multi-center Study on the Attitudes of Malaysian Emergency Health Care Staff towards Allowing Family Presence During Resuscitation of Adult Patients.' *International Journal of Emergency Medicine* 3 (2010): 287–91.

Spiro, H.M., M.G. McCrea Curnen and L.P. Wandel, eds. *Facing Death: Where Culture, Religion and Medicine Meet.* New Haven, CT: Yale University Press, 1996.

Theivendran, J. *House MD: An Analysis of Chronic Pain Managed with Opiate Therapy in Entertainment Television.* London: Imperial College Medical School, 2007.

Timmermans, S. 'Resuscitation Technology in The Emergency Department: Towards a Dignified Death.' *Sociol Health Illness* 20, no. 2 (1998): 144–67.

Timmermans, S. *Sudden Death and the Myth of CPR*, 1st edn. Philadelphia, PA: Temple University Press, 1999.

Tsai, E. 'Should Family Members Be Present During Cardiopulmonary Resuscitation?' *New England Journal Medicine* 346, no. 13 (2002): 1019–21.

Turow, J. 'Television Entertainment and the US Health-care Debate.' *Lancet* 347 (1996): 1240–3.

Turow, J. *Playing Doctor: Television, Storytelling, & Medical Power*, 2nd edn. Ann Arbor, MI: The University of Michigan Press, 2010.

Van Den Bulck, J. and K. Damiaans. 'Cardiopulmonary resuscitation on Flemish television: Challenges to the television effects Hypothesis.' *Emergency Medicine Journal* 21, no. 5 (2004): 565–7.

Wacht, O. 'The Attitudes of the Emergency Department Staff Toward Family Presence During Resuscitation.' M.H.A, Health Systems Management. Beer-Sheva: Ben- Gurion University of the Negev, 2008.

Wacht, O., K. Dopelt, Y. Snir and N. Davidovitch. 'Attitudes of Emergency Department Staff toward Family Presence During Resuscitation.' *The Israel Medicine Association Journal* 12, no. 6 (2010): 366–70.

Wallack E.M. and G.J. Bingle. 'Correspondence—Cardiopulmonary Resuscitation on Television. *New England Journal of Medicine* 335, no. 21 (1996): 1605–13.

## CHAPTER 3

# The *ER* Effect: How Medical Television Creates Knowledge for American Audiences

*Jessica Bodoh-Creed*

Americans have access to many forms of media that propel information toward audiences. They become passive consumers of this information, casually flipping through a magazine or watching television while eating dinner. According to Gerbner, 'In the typical U.S. home the television set is in use for more than seven hours a day,'[1] and we watch about five hours of television programming a day.[2] While television contains a vast array of programming options from fictional narrative stories to non-fictional news-based shows, 'television content ... influences mass culture because it provides widely shared common knowledge, beliefs and expectations.'[3] This research explores the fundamental shift in American public culture after the premiere of *ER*, a fictional medical television show, in 1994. With this shift, 'many Americans gain their medical and health information not from their physician or the medical profession but from the media.'[4]

While television is a central force in cultural change, outside social processes such as neoliberalism and biomedicalisation also contribute

J. Bodoh-Creed (✉)
Department of Anthropology, California State University, Los Angeles, CA, USA
e-mail: jessanthro@gmail.com

© The Author(s) 2017
E. Kendal and B. Diug (eds.), *Teaching Medicine and Medical Ethics Using Popular Culture*, Palgrave Studies in Science and Popular Culture, DOI 10.1007/978-3-319-65451-5_3

enormously to the circulation of information. David Harvey's work shows that 'Neoliberalism has, in short, become hegemonic as a mode of discourse. It has pervasive effects on ways of thought to the point where it has become incorporated into the common-sense way many of us interpret, live in, and understand the world.'[5] The social principles that come with the larger, more visible, political and economic framework often go unquestioned. The job then is to see how 'American neo-liberalism [functions] as a principle of intelligibility and a principle of decipherment of social relationships and individual behavior.'[6] The medical knowledge and healthy behaviours demonstrated in spaces such as media follow the guiding principles of neoliberal deregulation, freedom, personal responsibility and individuality that are openly encouraged of consumers. Neoliberalism has encouraged the public to become 'smart patients' on their own, by doing their own research and information gathering, and has contributed to the role of media within the knowledge audiences consume about biomedicine. Biomedicine is deeply connected to American culture and is creating ways for people to understand their own bodies and the world around them on a biological basis, from germs to viruses to organs and systems. Television is central to this healthscape of 'things medical,' which Clarke demonstrates through similar visual imagery and multiple media-based health information sources.[7] The media culture in which we exist creates new forms of information, often through images and a reliance on visual metaphors:

> Even as television portrays fictionalized, dramatized images of the existing medical culture, its choice of what to portray—and not to portray—simultaneously helps shape public perceptions of medicine that are carried into the clinic and the hospital by patients.[8]

It is the television writers, Hollywood television studios, the physicians and nurses working television who become the storytellers and information sources. For medical fictional television, the most important roles that are driving the creation of accurate medical knowledge are the physicians and nurses who write, advise and create the medicine on screen for viewers.

Clarke argues that 'in deeply significant but largely ignored ways, contemporary American biomedicalization itself is imbricated with popular and visual cultural materials, representations, and media coverage of things medical.'[7] These images and imagery of 'things medical' give perspective and grounding for patients or soon-to-be patients to better understand the biomedical world. This process is seen in medical fictional television where physician writers share their own stories from their medical practice that are then performed on screen: 'Both television and medicine ... became part and parcel of everyday living—integrated, naturalized, coconstitutive—during the deeply transformative medicalization healthscape.'[7] As media was creating a space for broader medical knowledge among audiences, biological citizenship and 'smart patients' were being encouraged by broader neoliberal social and cultural practices.[9] This research shows how medical television, especially after 1994 and the beginning of the run of the show *ER*, changed the landscape of medical information for American audiences. I propose that there is a process called the *ER* Effect, similar to the *CSI* Effect, whereby the show *ER* created a working medical imaginary and visual imagery that increased the flow of medical information for audiences.

## METHODS

This research employs a method called 'studying up,' whereby the people being sought for information are in a more privileged position than the researcher and do not have an obligation to speak with anyone about anything.[10,11] I chose to pursue this project that required engagement from the entertainment industry, although it could be an obstacle to traditional participant observation as an anthropological methodology. I acknowledge that I am in a privileged position because I began my work with industry informants by first connecting with an Executive Producer for *Grey's Anatomy* whom I knew personally, and this person led me to my first key informants. From there I utilised my current location of Los Angeles and the many friends I have working in the entertainment industry to find more informants. As I met more people, I gained an increasing legitimacy with informants who accepted that I was undertaking academic research, and not a super-fan or someone looking to meet famous people and get on set. One Executive Producer of several medical shows even stated that I knew some of the details of his shows better than he did, a clear case of academic study and not a casual viewer or fan.

Beginning in 2011, I spoke to many physicians, television medical writers, television medical technical advisors, product placement facilitators, actors who played doctors on television shows, and medical television producers and directors. Collectively they total about 100 people who work and have worked on shows such as *ER*, *St. Elsewhere*, *M\*A\*S\*H*, *Grey's Anatomy*, *Combat Hospital*, *Chicago Hope*, *Bones*, *Private Practice*, House, *M.D.*, Nip/*Tuck*, Doogie Howser, *M.D.*, Trapper John, *M.D.*, *Ben Casey*, *Scrubs*, *Monday Mornings*, and many other shows that are non-medical but have occasional medical storylines, in addition to countless commercials and feature films. I visited two television sets, one with a medical advisor on a non-medical show and a second with producers to a specifically medical show. These methods were supplemented with scattered pieces of research from a multitude of other sites.

## The *CSI* Effect

We often question how much viewers actually learn from television shows. One of the best examples with which we may compare medical television is legal television; these are close associates in television programming as they are both understood as 'procedural dramas.'[12] Anthropologist Laura Nader, writing in 1969, wrote that 'most of what we learn about the law we absorb vicariously from TV westerns and Perry Mason-style shows,' and the same is true today for medicine and other fields.[11] More recently, many scholars and prosecutors have cited something called the '*CSI* Effect' to discuss the effect of forensic shows on real life legal juries. In questioning what the *CSI* Effect is or means for legal cases, 'prosecutors claim that the show makes juries less inclined to convict because they have inflated expectations for the comprehensiveness, sophistication and clarity of forensic evidence–all those threads and fibers and DNA traces left behind at crime scenes.'[13] Audiences that watch the forensic or medical–legal show *CSI: Crime Scene Investigation*, on air since 2000 and with many spin-offs, have purportedly been paying close attention to the use of DNA testing, crime scene collection and other forensic processes in their television storylines.

Many medical, legal and forensic shows have been developed since, with shows such as *Bones*, *Dexter*, *Body of Proof*, *NCIS* and others, and even procedural legal shows such as *Law & Order* use forensic evidence prominently in their storylines. The medical examiners, pathologists and forensic scientists are major characters with laboratories full of high-tech equipment and fancy techniques to quickly find a clue the killer left behind that will put them behind bars. On *CSI* witnesses and humans lie, but science does not. These medical-legal shows are usually procedural, where the pattern of the episodes' story will be repetitive and the episodes are similar to one another (*House, M.D.*, a medical show, fits this pattern as well). On a procedural show, there is a crime committed, often a murder or almost deadly assault, and then the crime scene is mined for any and all evidence that may remain. That evidence is then carefully brought back to some sort of crime laboratory and processed in machinery by trained technicians, while law enforcement do their work in tracking and identifying suspects. 'On the one hand, *CSI* is read by both experts and mass media as fictional and not relevant for nonfictional forensic science, but on the other hand, they are concerned that other, nonexpert viewers will (mis)understand nonfictional practices through the prism of *CSI*.'[14] The *CSI* Effect is a demonstrated outcome of media knowledge on consumers and audiences that can be borrowed for the field of medical television in much the same way this effect has been shown in legal shows.

Even if it is debatable how much information audiences are taking from the medical–legal shows such as *CSI*, it is clear that the general public is more knowledgeable than ever about forensic investigative tools such as the collection of fingerprints, hair, semen, sweat and other bodily traces that can link back to the individual who committed a crime. Shows such as *CSI* have demonstrated specialised technology—mass spectrometers, for example—to the public, and people are generally more aware of these kinds of evidence and their implications. A 'stupid criminal' now is someone who does not wear gloves or a mask or a condom, or is careless with their hairs, or does not clean up blood with bleach, ever mindful of the cracks or blood seepage. This is a vastly different perspective from just 10 or 20 years ago, because there is more information circulating about this thanks to the popularity of the medical–legal or legal shows. In this way, the same can be said about general medical shows where audiences know more about new and rare diseases or about treatments for conditions because of such exposure. Through studies about consumers' knowledge retention about medical procedures and disease information and in-depth research with the medical staff of television shows, I aim to show that the *CSI* Effect is similar to the knowledge development that occurs through similar medical programming, something I call the *ER* Effect. After the creation of the show *ER*, medical programming began a quest for more authenticity with accurate medical terminology, more physicians on staff than any medical shows that came before and graphic medicine presented at its finest.

Part of the reason the *CSI* Effect, and the echoing *ER* Effect, are so compelling for audiences is their integration into the narrative of television storytelling. Most of the writers, directors and actors I spoke with told me that at a basic level they were telling a story. It all came back to the story of the show or the episode: 'Stories connect people into collectivities, and they coordinate actions among people who share the expectation that life will unfold according to certain plots.'[15] These television plots become group or collective narratives that are appealing to people, both sick and healthy. A story 'is as common as air' and so it is a familiar and appealing context for the consumer.[16] The *ER* Effect is compelling because of the use of medical authenticity *and* the narrative of the characters in the storyline. We care about the medicine because it is happening to or around our favourite characters, and that is often why medical shows can seem like night-time soap operas, because everyone is in constant danger. The narrative is heightened when beloved characters are in a plane or helicopter crash, shot in the hospital or are diagnosed with cancer, and all of these storylines are easily found in both *ER* and *Grey's Anatomy*. By creating a world the audience will want to see and experience every week, medical television pulls us into another world and we experience it alongside the characters, enjoying every minute of their joy and disappointment. The narrative and drama also make it seem as if being a doctor or working in a hospital is constantly exciting.

## The *ER* Effect

I met many physicians and nurses who work on television sets, always trying to inform non-medical writers and crew about their world. They give writers options for diseases patients could have, they write in medical terminology dialogue, they position actors in an emergency room set, they demonstrate inserting intubation tubes, and they often dress in scrubs and surgical wear to appear in the scene as background actors. These writers and advisors know about the blogs that point out medical mistakes and told me about the emails and letters they get from overzealous medical students pointing out the impossibility of a particular disease presentation. One informant said that she will not compromise on the kinds of medical points that people at home could put to use, such as CPR: 'Someone at home could save Grandma with this information,' she said. They work hard to ensure a balance between the drama of the

story and the stretching of medical possibilities to achieve both an entertaining show and a fairly accurate portrayal of medicine. Physician writers
also make sure the medical problems of the patients match up to the cor-
rect doctors involved in the storyline on the more broad medical shows.
If someone comes into the emergency room in either *ER* or *Grey's
Anatomy* and the writers want specific doctors involved with that patient,
then the disease or condition needs to match their specialties. As I was
told, a cardiologist is not going to consult with the orthopaedic surgeon
on a broken arm. But they might if there had been a car accident and
there was blunt force trauma to the torso, as well as a broken arm; so
there are strategies for connecting physicians together in a team to treat
a patient with accuracy. Many of the physician writers expressed difficulties because they felt that accuracy was something everyone thought they
should be chasing but no one seemed to be able to define what it exactly
meant. If accuracy is simply a reference to medically accurate information then most medical television is accurate, because the storylines have
the potential to happen in real life. According to physician writers some
expectations for accuracy were unrealistic, because otherwise there would
be a limit on the diseases they could show and the stories would begin
to get very repetitive. *House, M.D.* is usually the exception, because the
show's entire focus is on the rare diseases of medicine. Dr House is the
Sherlock Holmes of medicine in popular culture, and this allows for the
constant stream of new and rare diseases to be accepted and enjoyed by
audiences without critique.

The foundational and often cited medical studies about television
viewing and education are based on CPR rates and HIV transmission,
both viewed as potential sites for misinformation that would concern public health. Treichler, citing the Centers for Disease Control
and Prevention (CDC), states that '88 percent of the American public
obtains health information from television.'[4] Specifically for the case of
*ER*, this show had more doctors on staff as both writers and consultants
than any show ever made before. *ER* was created by trained physician
Michael Crichton, also a popular science fiction writer, although I have
been told that the producers had more to do with the look and feel of
the show than Crichton, who only wrote the pilot. Because of this heavy
involvement by physicians, *ER* was situated as a medical authority on television and therefore often criticised by the medical establishment.

In a study reported in the *New England Journal of Medicine*,
researchers looked at television episodes with a keen interest in CPR

or cardiopulmonary resuscitation and survival rates. They assert that 'Patients learn about CPR from many sources, including physicians, family and friends, personal experience, and CPR courses, [but] in a number of studies ... patients report that they obtain much of their information from the media.'[17] With this basis, researchers found that

> Survival rates for CPR on these television programs were significantly higher than the highest rates reported in the literature [for real patients]. For short-term survival, the rate of success on television was 75 percent, as compared with 40 percent in the literature (P < 0.001), and for long-term survival (assuming that the patients on *ER* about whom no explicit information was given survived to discharge), the rate of success was 67 percent (40 patients survived) as compared with 30 percent (P < 0.001).[17]

The differential survival rate on television and in real life is statistically dramatic. One of the physicians I interviewed who writes for television said that as a practising Emergency Room physician in Los Angeles, he runs a code (where the patient is crashing and CPR is administered) so that 'patients' families know everything has been done.' He believes that patients' families need to see doctors doing the work even if they are unable to save their loved one. They are told on television that CPR is a life-saving treatment, one that more often than not works to bring a family member back to life.

> The portrayal of CPR and death on three popular television programs is misleading in a number of ways ... [These] television programs give a misleading impression about the kind of people most commonly given CPR. On television, children, teenagers, and young adults accounted for 65 percent of the patients given CPR. Of the total number of deaths on the programs, 83 percent were of nonelderly patients. In fact, cardiac arrest is much more common in the elderly than in children or young adults.[17]

Physicians who work in television agreed that most often it is not healthy, young people that are crashing in real life and need CPR. It is often the very sick and the elderly, and they will have a higher death rate. 'Rates of long-term survival after cardiac arrest as reported in the medical literature vary from 2 percent to 30 percent for arrests outside a hospital, and from 6.5 percent to 15 percent for arrests that take place inside a hospital.'[17] Most often the physicians I interviewed when asked about CPR portrayals on television talked about these facts, but that does not give enough drama for television narratives. The drama and accuracy also lies in the realistic portrayal of CPR techniques on screen, created by *ER*'s on-set physicians, which now looks as realistic as it can without actually being the technique that is used in real life. In reality CPR does a lot of damage to the body while trying to get the heart pumping again, often breaking ribs in the process. On *ER*, the actors playing doctors were instructed to place their hands on the sternum of the actor playing the patient but to rhythmically move their own body up and down, often using their legs if straddling the patient, which creates the illusion of force. In a rebuttal to Diem et al. in the *NEJM*, Dr Neal Baer, a writer and producer on *ER*, wrote that 'two physicians are among the staff of six writers on *ER* and each script is reviewed by a physician trained in emergency medicine. The writers try to present stories based on real-life patients but sometimes dramatize the events to garner high ratings.'[18] Baer told me in an interview that this study 'gave us pause' because 'if we want people to feel it is real, people are going to believe what you are writing ... and we have a responsibility.'

Generally medical demonstrations in a scene should always look as medically sound as possible and give the most realistic portrayal of medicine. A writer for *ER* talked extensively about the awards given to the show for its coverage of HIV/AIDS storylines and the publicity that resulted. Baer felt this storyline with the character of Jeanie Boulet was one of the most important they did on *ER* and 'dispelled myths about HIV' for the audience. Substance abuse for the Dr House character on *House, M.D.* was an example given by several writers for the show as their favourite and most important storyline. *Grey's Anatomy* featured a story about woman who had a preventative double mastectomy, and a writer for the show discussed how important that storyline was for the cast and crew. These stories are all good exposure for the shows and educational opportunities for the audience. Paired together, this is the *ER* Effect at its best. One medical advisor told me that she would have shows hire real amputees, actual children with cystic fibrosis and real survivors of chemotherapy as background actors when they were needed for hospital sets on various shows, and then those shows would get fantastic feedback from those communities about their portrayal. It was important for her to include the reality in the medicine in small ways like this, and her efforts resonated with audiences.

A Kaiser Family Foundation study of viewer responses and recall to an *ER* episode found that '53% of regular viewers say they learn about important health care issues from *ER*.'[19] Importantly, Americans seem to enjoy programming that they see as both informational and entertaining, so that *ER* was not only seen as realistic in its portrayal of medicine, but it also showed something that captured people's interest beyond just that. It was also noted that '62% of those who say they learn about health issues from *ER* also say that's one of the reasons they watch the show, including 25% who said it was a "major" reason they watched the show.'[19] Medical television has long had interactions with medical groups such as the American Medical Association and Los Angeles County Medical Association since the 1960s, and organisations such as Hollywood, Health & Society, funded by the CDC, USC, and NIH, more recently. Medical television chose early on to self-regulate, beginning in the 1960s with *City Hospital* and *Ben Casey*, and involves specialists such as doctors and nurses to make the medical process more real for audiences. The hospitals of *Ben Casey* in the 1960s look very different from *St. Elsewhere* in the 1980s, and extremely different from the hospitals from the 1990s to the present. The largest difference over this timeframe is the amount of machinery, blood and organs seen on screen, where television programs before *ER*, even shows such as *M\*A\*S\*H*, set in a war, do not show graphic injuries. A medical consultant and nurse who has worked in the industry longer than anyone else I have spoken with stated that when she looks back at the shows she worked on from the 1960s to the 1980s, the biggest transition has been in what you can show on screen now: 'We couldn't show blood [in the 1980s], no visible hearts [in a body cavity], but they wanted it to *look* real.' She was working in the era right before *ER*, and the shift in the 1990s was drastic for the television industry. Shows from the 2000s such as *Grey's Anatomy* and *House M.D.* have featured open fractures, open chest cavities, open skulls with brain exposed, open everything; bodies are now open to audiences in all their blood spurting, pulsing, need for medical attention.

I also spoke with an Executive Producer for *ER* who described the studio's hesitation over having a show that had such a vast amount of medical jargon as dialogue. This medical discourse posed a significant challenge for them, and the producers had to explain that not only did they think the television audience was ready for it, but that the studio should think of the 'medical language as like wallpaper. It's just there. It's the background.' They quickly proved that American viewers wanted that fast-paced, quick, specialised jargon, because 'The attraction of these programs [*ER*, *Chicago Hope* and *Rescue 911*] rests in their graphic "realism."'[20] There is an expectation that the medicine is real on these shows, and therefore the audience might pick up on the presented information, tendencies and terminology. The dramatically graphic and perceived realism on *ER* created a new medical imaginary for television, and the *ER* Effect. Within that frame, *ER* gave audiences at home the feeling they were getting an inside and a 'real' look at an actual emergency room.

The *ER* Effect demonstrates the movement of traditional medical knowledge to audiences who received it from this unusual source. When patients go into their doctor's office quoting *Dr. Oz* or *ER*, it is not always treated as expert knowledge because of the processes of translation through the show, but this is becoming more and more common as the *ER* Effect has grown alongside the *CSI* Effect. This kind of real, traditional knowledge presented in fictional programming is usually based on the idea of edutainment or infotainment, the process of both entertaining and informing people at the same time, maybe so well that they do not even know that they are learning. Brodie et al. surveyed viewers about the *ER* storyline on HIV/AIDS between 1997 and 2000, and more than half stated they watch for health information as well as entertainment.[21] There is something that appeals to American audiences about enjoying the knowledge that is delivered to them via this programming. Brodie et al. note that 'About one in seven viewers said that they contacted their doctor or health care provider about a health problem because of something they saw on *ER*.'[24] The knowledge being produced on *ER* contributed to their own bodily health, their general health education, and it is a trend that has continued on in popular medical shows, including *House M.D.* and *Grey's Anatomy*.

A physician writer on *ER* told me about a viewer who contacted him after an episode of *ER* saved her life. The viewer had chronic headaches and was not getting answers from her physicians. In the episode, Dr Mark Greene (played by Anthony Edwards) is shown to have a recurrence of his brain tumour when he sticks out his tongue and it deviates to one side. This woman at home went to the mirror and stuck out her tongue. It deviated left as well, and when she immediately went to the emergency room she was diagnosed with a tumour behind her nose. Doctors said she would have died within a few weeks if they had not caught it. She went through chemotherapy and surgery, and is still alive today, ten years later. The woman contacted the physician writer, and he flew her out to Los Angeles to tour the set of *ER* and meet everyone. She still calls this writer her 'angel.' This is the *ER* Effect at its best.

## CONCLUSION

One of the forensic consultants for medical–legal shows (both fictional and reality television) told me that in her opinion the *CSI* Effect 'is slightly overrated but definitely exists' and that '*CSI* is more technology driven than a lot of other shows' where character storylines draw away from such a technology-heavy focus. The consultant went on to say that the 'technology is ridiculous' and 'if all that worked, there would be no need for actual people.'[25] There are holograms, wildly accurate photo mapping, pixelating and facial recognition computer programs that can be seen on medical–legal or legal–police procedural shows, but do not exist in real life. In stark contrast, almost all of the technology and medical procedures are real on medical shows, which may lead to more accurate understanding by audiences from the *ER* Effect. Shows such as *Grey's Anatomy* work to include the newest technological and scientific advances in their episodes, for example an episode featuring the 'Heart in a Box' device, which the show secured from the man who designed the device directly after Food and Drug Administration (FDA) approval.[22] In this way, the *ER* Effect is more effective at passing along accurate and authentic information to audiences, more so than the *CSI* type shows with fictional technologies.

The *ER* Effect is produced by members of the medical and television community who have taken it upon themselves to self-regulate in order to ensure public health and safety messages are clear and authentic. The doctors and nurses who work on shows, especially since the era of *ER*, push for more realistic portrayals of patients, medicine and disease when depicting brain surgery or heart attacks. This effect from *ER* has left lasting impressions in television production values and subsequently on viewers. When a viewer sees Dr Oz holding up a lung, as he is wont to do, it is probably not the first lung they think they have ever seen. They perhaps saw a pig lung or a modelled silicone lung on a fictional medical show long before Dr Oz was making viewers put on gloves and hold them. *ER* changed the medical landscape for television, introducing audiences to complicated jargon, bloody gowns and rushing around the emergency room. One of the writer/producers of *ER* told me that he did not personally know what 'bradying down' meant, even though he had written it into hundreds of *ER* scripts. When this writer was in the hospital with a sick family member and heard that phrase 'the patient is bradying down,' he called for help in the hallway because the only thing he knew was 'that was what I put in scripts when things weren't going well with the patient, so I only knew it was really bad.' Even the non-medical writers gained medical information via the *ER* Effect from working on the show. Incidentally, 'bradying down' means that the heart rate of the patient is dangerously slow.

The *ER* Effect ripples not only through the audience, but also through the medical community. Two physicians who worked on *ER* said that applications for medical school went up during *ER*'s highest ratings years, as did the selection of emergency medicine as a specialty; anecdotally, one had heard a rate of over 300%. I spoke to one physician who consulted on a show because of the specific nature of their specialty who told me that if potential physicians are 'getting a sense of how to behave [as a doctor] from TV, they should not be in medicine,' but that people at home wanted to do what the doctors on *ER* did. It has also been reported that 'For their most obvious stabs at realism the creators of both *ER* and *Chicago Hope* turned to the kind of gore and frankness about illnesses that a few years before several people in Hollywood confidently stated that the audience wouldn't accept.'[23] The 'gore' or medically graphic presentation of bodies, diseased and injured bodies, was a larger social phenomenon. The level of graphic realism and this change over time towards more realistic presentation is exemplary of Clarke's visual imagery realised as 'things medical,' whereby audiences began to be interested about what the inside of bodies look like and what physicians really see when patients have been shot or stabbed and come into an emergency room.[7] I interviewed Noah Wyle (Dr John Carter on *ER*) after a physician writer for the show described him as one of the actors most interested in the medicine on *ER*. Wyle told me that early in the run of *ER* his friends would come over to his house and find 'frankenchickens' in his freezer that he used to practise suturing. He, along with other cast members, did 'ride alongs' where they shadowed real emergency room physicians; he read medical textbooks, anatomy and physiology texts, and diaries of medical students to familiarise himself with what life would really be like as an intern. Wyle also admitted that he was ambitious, hungry and 'grew to love the seal of approval from the medical community' conferred upon *ER*.

One of the major criticisms of *ER* and several other medical shows was the lack of industry accuracy with respect to the role of interns and residents. There are claims that '[*ER*] has paid lip service to med ed's "see one, do one, teach one" method ... [but] naysayers point out [that in real life] a third-year would never be dispatched to do half the procedures that Carter [on *ER*] gets to do on his own.'[24] Physician writers discussed having committed those medical errors, but for the sake of the storyline. It adds urgency and fear if someone who seems inexperienced is left with the responsibility of saving a life, and when they save someone there is a bigger pay off for the audience and the character. These issues of authenticity and accuracy were raised with my informants often, but they believe that these are negligible and necessary for the drama of the episodes.

Television provides a medical imaginary of what can and should be for bodies within biomedicine: 'The mass media ... present a rich, ever-changing store of possible lives, some of which enter the lived imaginations of ordinary people more successfully than others.'[25] Medical narratives and stories are that of life and death, they are scary and uplifting, they make viewers cry and laugh, and these stories are written and set up by physicians and nurses who want them to be better and more accurate. The *ER* Effect demonstrates a crucial transition in medical television whereby when people learn from this kind of graphic, real television, they see something that will shape their biomedical perception.

## Notes

1. G. Gerbner, 'Cultivation Analysis: An Overview,' *Mass Communication and Society* 1, no. 3/4 (1998): 175–94.
2. B. Stelter, 'Neilsen Reports Decline in Television Viewing,' *The New York Times*, 3 May 2012.
3. C.P. Kottak, *Prime-Time Society: An Anthropological Analysis of Television and Culture* (Belmont, CA: Wadsworth Publishing Company, 1990).
4. P. Treichler, 'Medicine, Popular Culture and the Power of Narrative: The HIV/AIDS Storyline on General Hospital,' in *Medicine's Moving Pictures*, ed. L. Reagan, N. Tomes and P.A. Treichler (Rochester, NY: University of Rochester Press, 2007) 93–132.
5. D. Harvey, *A Brief History of Neoliberalism* (Oxford: Oxford University Press, 2005).
6. M. Foucault, *The Birth of Biopolitics: Lectures at the College Dr France 1978–79*, Ed. M. Senellart (New York: Palgrave Macmillan, 2008).

7. A.E. Clarke, 'The Rise of Medicine to Biomedicalization: U.S. Healthscapes and Iconography, Circa 1890–Present,' in *Biomedicalization: Technoscience, Health, and Illness in the U.S.*, ed. A.E. Clarke, L. Mamo, J.R. Fosket, J.R. Fishman and J.K. Shim (Durham, NC: Duke University Press, 2010), 104–46.

8. G, Vandekieft, 'From *City Hospital* to *ER*: The Evolution of the Television Physician,' in *Cultural Sutures: Medicine and Media*, ed. L.D. Friedman (Durham, NC: Duke University Press, 2004), 215–33.

9. N. Rose, *The Politics of Life Itself: Biomedicine, Power, and Subjectivity in the Twenty-First Century* (Princeton, NJ: Princeton University Press, 2007).

10. H. Gusterson, 'Studying Up Revisited,' *Political and Legal Anthropology Review* 20, no. 1 (1997): 114–19.

11. L. Nader, 'Up the Anthropologist—Perspectives Gained From Studying Up,' in *Reinventing Anthropology*, ed. D. Hymes (New York: Pantheon Books, 1969), 284–311.

12. C. Harris, 'The Evidence Doesn't Lie: Genre Literacy and the CSI Effect,' *Journal of Popular Film and Television* 29, no. 1 (2011): 2–11.

13. S. Cole and R. Dioso, 'Law and the Lab: Do TV Shows Really Affect How Juries Vote? Let's Look at the Evidence,' *Wall Street Journal Online*, 2005.

14. C. Kruse, 'Producing Absolute Truth: *CSI* Science as Wishful Thinking,' *American Anthropologist* 112, no. 1 (2010): 79–91.

15. A.W. Frank, *Letting Stories Breathe: A Socio-Narrative* (Chicago: University of Chicago Press, 2010).

16. L.C. Garro and C. Mattingly, 'Narrative as Construct and Construction,' in *Narrative and the Cultural Construction of Healing and Illness*, ed. C. Mattingly and L.C. Garro (Berkeley: University of California Press, 2000), 1–49.

17. S.J. Diem, J.D. Lantos and J.A. Tulsky, 'Cardiopulmonary Resuscitation on Television: Miracles and Misinformation,' *New England Journal of Medicine* 334 (1996): 1578–82.

18. N. Baer, 'Cardiopulmonary Resuscitation on Television: Exaggerations and Accusations,' *New England Journal of Medicine*, 334 (1996): 1604–6.

19. Kaiser Family FoundationKaiser Family Foundation, 'Documenting the Power of Television – A Survey of Regular E.R. Viewers about Emergency Contraception – Summary of Findings' (2007), available at: http://kff.org/womens-health-policy/poll-finding/documenting-the-power-of-television-a-survey-2/.

20. S.E. Lederer and N. Rogers, 'Media,' in *Companion to Medicine in the Twentieth Century*, ed. R. Cooter and J. Pickstone (London: Routledge, 2003), 487–502.
21. M. Brodie, U. Foehr, V. Rideout, N. Baer, C. Miller, R. Flournoy and D. Altman, 'Communicating Health Information Through the Entertainment Media,' *Health Affairs* 20, no. 1 (2001): 192–9.
22. *Grey's Anatomy*, 'Heart-Shaped Box,' Season 8, Episode 8, Screened 3 November 2011 (United States of America: LIFE, 2011).
23. J. Turow, *Playing Doctor: Television, Storytelling, and Medical Power* (Ann Arbor: The University of Michigan Press, 2010).
24. C. Durso, 'Specialized Television,' *New Physician* 44, no. 1 (1995): 19–22.
25. A. Appadurai, *Modernity at Large: Cultural Dimensions of Globalization* (Minneapolis: University of Minnesota Press, 1996).

## BIBLIOGRAPHY

Appadurai, A. *Modernity at Large: Cultural Dimensions of Globalization.* Minneapolis: University of Minnesota Press, 1996.

Baer, N. 'Cardiopulmonary Resuscitation on Television: Exaggerations and Accusations.' *New England Journal of Medicine* 334 (1996): 1604–6.

Brodie, M., U. Foehr, V. Rideout, N. Baer, C. Miller, R. Flournoy and D. Altman. 'Communicating Health Information Through the Entertainment Media.' *Health Affairs* 20, no.1 (2001): 192–9.

Clarke, A.E., L. Mamo, J.R. Fosket, J.R. Fishman and J.K. Shim, eds. *Biomedicalization: Technoscience, Health, and Illness in the U.S.* Durham, NC: Duke University Press, 2010.

Cole, S. and R. Dioso. 'Law and the Lab: Do TV Shows Really Affect How Juries Vote? Let's Look at the Evidence.' *Wall Street Journal Online*, 2005, available at: http://truthinjustice.org/law-lab.htm.

Cooter, R and J Pickstone, eds. *Companion to Medicine in the Twentieth Century.* London: Routledge, 2003.

Diem, S.J., J.D. Lantos and J.A. Tulsky. 'Cardiopulmonary Resuscitation on Television: Miracles and Misinformation.' *New England Journal of Medicine* 334 (1996): 1578–82.

Durso, C. 'Specialized Television.' *New Physician* 44, no. 1 (1995): 19–22.

Foucault, M. 'The Birth of Biopolitics: Lectures at the College Dr France 1978–79,' Ed. M. Senellart. New York: Palgrave Macmillan, 2008.

Frank, A.W. 'Letting Stories Breathe: A Socio-Narrative.' Chicago: University of Chicago Press, 2010.

Friedman, L.D., ed. *Cultural Sutures: Medicine and Media.* Durham, NC: Duke University Press, 2004.

Garro, L.C. and C. Mattingly, eds. *Narrative and the Cultural Construction of Healing and Illness*. Berkeley: University of California Press, 2000.

Gerbner, G. 'Cultivation Analysis: An Overview.' *Mass Communication and Society* 1 no. 3/4 (1998): 175–94.

Gusterson, H. 'Studying Up Revisited.' *Political and Legal Anthropology Review* 20, no. 1 (1997): 114–9.

Harvey, D. *A Brief History of Neoliberalism*. Oxford: Oxford University Press, 2005.

Hymes, D. Ed. *Reinventing Anthropology*. New York: Pantheon Books, 1969.

Kaiser Family Foundation. 'Documenting the Power of Television—A Survey of Regular E.R. Viewers about Emergency Contraception—Summary of Findings,' 2007, available at: http://kff.org/womens-health-policy/poll-finding/documenting-the-power-of-television-a-survey-2/. Accessed 7 June 2013.

Kottak, C.P. 'Prime-Time Society: An Anthropological Analysis of Television and Culture.' Belmont, CA: Wadsworth Publishing Company, 1990.

Kruse, C. 'Producing Absolute Truth: *CSI* Science as Wishful Thinking.' *American Anthropologist* 112, no. 1 (2010): 79–91.

Reagan, L., N. Tomes and P.A. Treichler, eds. *Medicine's Moving Pictures*. Rochester, NY: University of Rochester Press, 2007.

Rose, N. *The Politics of Life Itself: Biomedicine, Power, and Subjectivity in the Twenty-First Century*. Princeton, NJ: Princeton University Press, 2007.

Stelter, B. 'Neilsen Reports Decline in Television Viewing,' *The New York Times*, New York, [Internet] 3 May 2012, [cited 26 August 2015], available at: http://mediadecoder.blogs.nytimes.com/2012/05/03/nielsen-reports-a-decline-in-television-viewing/?_r=0.

Turow, J. *Playing Doctor: Television, Storytelling, and Medical Power*, New and Expanded Ed. Ann Arbor: The University of Michigan Press, 2010.

## CHAPTER 4

# WhyZombie? Zombie Pop Culture to Improve Infection Prevention and Control Practices

*Peta-Anne Zimmerman and Matt Mason*

Throughout history humans have been fascinated and disgusted by the idea of corpses being reanimated and becoming the walking dead, or zombies. Historically, this dates back to the eighth century, presenting as fables, part of ancient myth and lore, that explore ontological anxieties.[1] They are stories of horror that warn humanity to heed their place in the universe and their role in maintaining balance of the Earth; spiritually, culturally and biologically.[2] These tales often warn against the desire to meddle with the fabric of the universe, or to bear the potentially apocalyptic consequences of such actions. The idea of the walking dead, or zombies, has therefore remained a constant in popular culture.

P.-A. Zimmerman (✉)
Griffith University, School of Nursing and Midwifery, Southport,
Queensland, Australia
e-mail: p.zimmerman@griffith.edu.au

M. Mason
University of the Sunshine Coast, Maroochydore DC,
Queensland, Australia
e-mail: mmason1@usc.edu.au

© The Author(s) 2017
E. Kendal and B. Diug (eds.), *Teaching Medicine and Medical Ethics Using Popular Culture*, Palgrave Studies in Science and Popular Culture, DOI 10.1007/978-3-319-65451-5_4

Popular culture and urban mythology are known methods for educating and training individuals in a number of fields. Whether supernatural or science fiction themed, the use of pop-cultural references can enhance the learning experience for individuals and groups as a whole.[3] Popular culture has, throughout history, initiated innovation that has led to science fiction becoming science fact. It was not so long ago that Aldous Huxley was describing a 'Brave New World,' Isaac Asimov was writing the first law of robotics and Gene Roddenberry and the *Star Trek* team were introducing viewers to what are now called tele-conferencing, mobile phones and tablets. Are we very far off from having 'tricorders' as a diagnostic instrument for medicine with our use of handheld thermal scanners?

## Traditional Infection Prevention and Control Education

Infection prevention and control is a key aspect of all undergraduate health professions and the delivery of patient care. It contributes to both patient and healthcare worker safety and is recognised as a global priority by the World Health Organization (WHO) and its member states, including Australia, with the First Global Patient Safety Challenge, Clean Care is Safer Care, launched in 2005.[4] An important part of this initiative is the education and training of healthcare workers in infection prevention and control.

Infection prevention and control education is, however, notoriously 'vanilla,' in the sense that it mainly consists of annual staff training, in-service programmes, posters, reporting of audit results and online learning. Generally speaking, it is considered a chore and little attention is paid by healthcare workers. Allen, Currey and Considine state that 'Assessment must not be undertaken simply for the purpose of assessment. When used, assessment must contribute to the learning experience—i.e. be conducted *for* and *of* learning,' which is often not the case in practice where staff undertake annual competencies, increasingly in an online format, purely to meet an administrative requirement.[5] It is for this reason perhaps that there are approximately 200,000 healthcare associated infections reported each year from Australian health facilities, which makes them the most common complication for patients.[6] Even with these statistics well known, the situation remains that standard and transmission-based precautions are still not well complied with by health-care workers.[7]

The literature, and healthcare history abounds with examples of how infection prevention and control is not done, of which the most recent Ebola virus disease (EVD) outbreak in West Africa and the percolating Middle East Respiratory Syndrome (MERs) are examples.[8] Before that, Severe Acute Respiratory Syndrome (SARS), the highly pathogenic avian influenzas, followed similar patterns. All of these infectious diseases have been amplified in the healthcare setting, primarily because of poor everyday infection prevention and control practice, and poor identification of infectious diseases. The challenge for healthcare educators is to make the content accessible, palatable and memorable to facilitate knowledge translating to practice.

## Pop-Culture Pedagogy

Pop culture as a pedagogical device uses content with which people are familiar, generally through film and television, in order to teach. It uses what has been described as the 'self-referential effect,' where an individual can relate to an idea or concept because they have lived it either physically or in their mind by processing a story.[9] Once the viewer makes a personal identification with an idea or concept they remember and can contextualise it. This is dependent upon the target audience and the pop-cultural references that they will respond to, as not all people have the same exposure or experience with popular culture. However, it remains that using such devices encourages active learning, corrects misconceptions, instils greater self-confidence and provides a better understanding of concepts.

Research indicates that pop-cultural references, such as storylines in film, television and literature, have a significant impact on audiences.[10] There are a number of narratives in the literature that explore the impact of popular culture on society and how that can then be best used to affect change or even rally awareness. The video game *Resident Evil 2* has been used to make parallels with the state of global health and security and the totalitarian state.[11] The commentary on 'witchcraft science' by Foreman expresses the concern that the medicine and science presented in popular media is distorted and clearly not a true representation of healthcare, though the public remember and cling to these depictions.[12] This has been demonstrated by a study that ascertained that young adults in particular gain their knowledge about HIV, amongst other sexually transmitted infections, through what they view on television.[13] It is therefore evident that the narratives and stories to which the general public are exposed, including those who are healthcare workers, can also be used as devices to influence and potentially change behaviour.

## WHY ZOMBIE?

So, why are zombies a good teaching device for improving infection prevention and control practice?

It all started with a Twitter conversation, when the question 'What is your favourite movie with an infectious disease cause?' was asked. One respondent cited *Shaun of the Dead*, which created an avalanche of zombie film suggestions. Another respondent then suggested that these films did not count as examples of 'infectious disease,' but we and others argued differently, citing the many films that did indeed have a pathogenic cause for 'zombification.' Buoyed by the idea that a number of us working in infection control were also pop-culture geeks, we thought some research was in order.

McCullough, in the seminal and very useful work, *Zombies: A Hunter's Guide*, identifies five main types of zombies:[14]

- Necromantic (raised from the grave by sorcery);
- Voodoo (black magic);
- Nazi zombies (necromancy ordered by Hitler);
- Revenants (return from the grave with revenge on their mind);
- Atomic (radiation exposure).

Even with these types identified, McCullough also identifies pathogenic sources as important in zombie activity, which is supported by Brooks, Munz et al. and Montandon.[15]

Wikipedia listed 383 feature-length 'A-list' zombie films, released between 1932 and 2014.[16] These films indicated a number of causes of 'zombification,' including microbial agents that have not been contained and spread readily from person to person. We further searched English language feature-length films, released from 2000 to 2014. Each film was checked against the publicly available databases IMDb, Rotten Tomatoes and Wikipedia to identify the cause of the zombie infestation featured in each film.

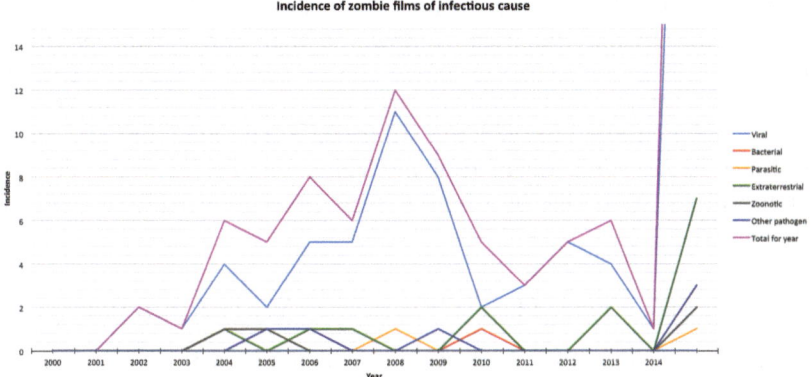

**Fig. 4.1**  Incidence of zombie films of infectious cause

On review of the films included on the Wikipedia list, 238 zombie films were released from 2000 to 2014.[17] Of these, 69 films had an infectious cause of some kind (viral, bacterial, parasite, extra-terrestrial, zoonotic or other biological cause). For 48 films the cause was unclear. In the remainder (n = 121), 'zombification' had no traceable infectious cause. When looking at release dates we realised there was a possible link between 'zombification' cause and global health events.

To test our hypothesis, we mapped the year of release of pathogenic zombie films against the World Health Organization's list of infectious disease outbreaks as seen in Fig. 4.1.[18] This demonstrated a correlation between the two, with an increase in the release of infectious biohorror films in the years following outbreaks such as SARS and pandemic influenza. So it appeared that global health threats have an impact on pop-culture media. This is also reported in the literature, where horror films are identified as a barometer of society's fears, anxieties and cultural consciousness.[19]

To provide more insight into this, British zombie film maker, Anthony D. Lane, currently producing and directing *Invasion of the Not Quite Dead* (due for release in 2017) stated, 'It [global outbreaks] definitely has an impact on our films. Our latest film is about an infectious disease that escapes from a lab and causes an outbreak in the town.'[20]

The zombie phenomenon has also been used by the United States Centers for Disease Control and Prevention (CDC) as a promotional device for public health preparedness and response.[21] The United States Strategic Command has used zombies to train junior officers citing: 'Using this fictitious scenario avoided concerns over the use of classified information, it resolved sensitivity to using real-world nations or scenarios, and it better engaged the students.'[22] The literature also demonstrates its use in mathematical modelling for disease outbreaks and for use in raising public health awareness, prevention and containment strategies.[23]

## IN THE CROSS-HAIRS: TARGETING YOUR AUDIENCE

So, how might educators best make use of these relationships to teach healthcare workers about safe infection prevention and control practice?

First, it is important to pick your audience and match the images to their sensibilities. While the Traffic Accident Commission of Victoria has proven since the late 1980s that there is a role in confronting an audience, zombies are not for everyone and we need to be mindful that we do not turn people away from the message through the images we choose to use.[24] When choosing clips or images, teachers may find that groups of extroverts (such as nurses from the Emergency Department) are more likely to engage with zombie references than others. However, this is a generalisation and the individual teacher will need to ascertain the level of acceptance within their intended audience. Providing a warning about graphic content before starting your session is advisable.

If the teacher identifies that the group may be put off by a zombie-themed learning experience, the opportunity to use pop-culture pedagogy should not be abandoned. Amul Mattu presented an overview of how a successful career in emergency medicine can be achieved by exploring the principles espoused in the film *The Princess Bride* at the popular Social Media And Critical Care (SMACC) conference, which regularly employs innovative pedagogy in critical care education.[25] This type of presentation can be used as a gateway to presenting more confrontational material and as a gauge to audience acceptance of this mode of learning.

## CRICKET BATS OR CROSSBOWS: THE DELIVERY

Once the audience is identified the teacher may select images/clips that illustrate the salient points. Zombie films, *World War Z* being an exception, tend not to be box office smashes so they are also unlikely to be well known outside those with an interest in the genre. Because of this, teachers cannot count on subtext within the film to be known and therefore need to choose images/clips that are unambiguous and clearly linked to the message conveyed in the class. Another issue to consider is that many of these films will be low budget and possibly low in quality, which may reflect on the presentation. Films such as *Shaun of the Dead* and *28 Days Later* offer high-quality production values and a range of scenes, and can therefore be used to advocate for more rigorous infection prevention and control practice.[26] Examples that we have used previously include a scene from *Shaun of the Dead* to highlight the use of personal protective equipment (PPE) in trauma settings and a scene from the Australian movie *Undead* that champions the role of the infection prevention and control professional.[27]

Capturing the images/clips is not particularly difficult, but educators should be aware of copyright laws relevant to their jurisdiction. Many of the more popular scenes/films are available on YouTube, which has a facility to embed the selected clip within a PowerPoint presentation. This also includes an option to embed a trimmed clip so that you are only including the parts of the movie you want to show. If you are feeling a little more adventurous it is possible, and a lot of fun, to make your own clip. This is particularly engaging if you get staff involved and adds to the reinforcement of the message. Making a short clip can be done cheaply through the use of a smartphone or digital camera and editing software such as Windows Movie Maker. Again, YouTube is a great resource here, with many videos being available to help you through the technical aspects of doing this.

## TEAM Z IN ACTION

What is the experience of actually using zombie pop culture as a pedagogical tool?

There are many examples of zombie scenarios being used to improve practice in healthcare. The following two show how the authors used a fictional situation to bring forth a discussion regarding contemporary nursing practice. Stanley provides nurses with an overview of how to prepare for an impending zombie apocalypse.[28] The focus of this is on developing the ability of nurses to recognise and respond to Solanum infection, in particular the required initial (recognition and isolation) and secondary nursing interventions (dealing with reanimation, palliative care and psychological support). The author's suggestion that a zombie epidemic is theoretically possible may seem far fetched, yet the fact remains that nurses in particular are responsible for implementing many initial and secondary interventions in any outbreak of disease.[29] These would include isolation/quarantine and infection prevention, observations, medication administration and other interventions, all of which put the nurse/healthcare worker at some risk.

Reinforcing this message is an article by Lowe and Hummel that uses the CDC resources to educate nurses on the role they play in disaster preparedness.[30] This article not only includes references to workplace health and safety, but also to personal preparedness at home. Personal preparedness is often overlooked, with health services expecting full attendance by staff when in fact this can be severely limited as staff may be injured/dead, unable to access the health service or are required to provide care for their family.[31]

Brooks highlights the need to be prepared in the event of a zombie outbreak and suggests that avoiding places of high zombie populations (hospitals for instance) is safer.[32] Interestingly, Brooks also points out that hospitals are potentially the worst place to head to in the event of a zombie apocalypse, as up to 90% of first-wave zombies tend to be healthcare workers exposed because of poor disease identification and infection prevention practices, such as not recognising potentially infected individuals at triage.[33] For those planning for disasters in healthcare this is an important point to note, and while in more common disasters hospitals do tend to be safer they are not without risk. Cassir et al. and Tomas et al. show the role of contaminated PPE in potentially spreading disease owing to poor doffing procedures.[34] This is an area highly suited to using zombie scenarios in training. The outbreaks of SARS, MERs and Ebola showed that health services can be a centre of amplification of outbreaks. Knowing this can temper the enthusiasm of staff to attend work during outbreaks, particularly if training and planning have not specifically addressed these concerns.

Our own experience as educators and infection prevention and control specialists has been to recently challenge our own colleagues to reinvigorate their education programmes and think outside the box. At the 2014 Australasian College for Infection Prevention Control (ACIPC) Conference, we presented our theory of using pop culture as a method to teach the basics of infection prevention and control. The scenes described above demonstrated the applicability of the genre to both standard and transmission-based precautions. What else can better demonstrate the need for personal protective equipment than the use of a cricket bat to incapacitate a zombie and the resulting blood splatter that ensues? Our colleagues agreed, and considered it to be a novel way to get their point across—particularly in the Emergency Department.

We currently employ pop culture in our own teaching, not only zombies, but also superheroes (*Spiderman* is arguably the result of zoonotic transmission), television shows (if you want to learn about Creutzfeldt Jakob disease watch the *X-Files*), popular games (*Resident Evil 2*) or contemporary literature (real vampires do not sparkle, but are a good example of poor standard precautions). As trained Global Outbreak Alert and Response Network (GOARN) members, we employ it to train others, with a video currently in production to support training of healthcare workers in the rapid identification and implementation of appropriate infection prevention and control precautions for a previously unknown infectious disease. The protagonist may have recently provided first aid to a person who collapsed in the street, who had profuse bleeding from their mouth and was coughing. This person scratched our hero. The collapsed person ... may have been living near a lab ... that may have exploded ... which caused an odd dust cloud ... which everyone in a one kilometre radius may have inhaled. You can make up the rest.

## Conclusion

The ease with which pop-culture references can be incorporated into educational and/or awareness campaigns is evident, as is the success factor for participants remembering what they have actually learned. When it comes to our specialty, zombies are a natural conduit for educating about emerging infectious diseases and the importance of infection prevention and control practices. Recurring themes in films that can be adapted to provide case studies include unknown transmission routes; appropriate use of PPE; quarantine and isolation and identifying and managing personal exposure. This method is not just limited to traditional methods of educational delivery: smartphones, applications, games, online learning packages and team-building exercises all offer the opportunity for immersive learning.

The sky really is the limit, but just be careful: that sky could contain highly pathogenic extra-terrestrial zombie-causing disease.

## Notes

1. 'History of Zombies,' 2016, available at: http://anthropology.msu.edu/anp264-ss13/2013/04/25/history-of-zombies/; Kevin Alexander Boon, 'Ontological Anxiety Made Flesh: The Zombie in Literature, Film and Culture,' in *Monsters and the Monstrous: Myths and Metaphors of Enduring Evil*, ed. Niall Scott (Amsterdam: Rodopi, 2007), 33–44.
2. Kline, Jim, 'Zombie Typology,' *Psychological Perspectives* 55 (2012): 467–81.
3. H. Jenkins, R. Purushotma, M. Weigel, K. Clinton and A.J. Robinson, *Confronting the Challenges of Participatory Culture: Media Education for the 21st Century* (Cambridge, MA: MIT Press, 2009).
4. World Health Organization, *WHO: Clean Care is Safer Care* (2005), available at: http://www.who.int/gpsc/en/.
5. J.A. Allen, J. Currey and J. Considine, 'Annual Resuscitation Competency Assessments: A Review of the Evidence,' *Australian Critical Care: Official Journal of the Confederation of Australian Critical Care Nurses* 26, no. 1 (2013): 12–7.
6. Clinical Excellence Commission, *Healthcare Associated Infections Program* (2015), available at: http://www.cec.health.nsw.gov.au/programs/hai.
7. National Health and Medical Research Council, *Australian Guidelines for the Prevention and Control of Infection in Healthcare*, (Canberra: Commonwealth of Australia, 2010), available at: http://www.legislationreview.nhmrc.gov.au/_files_nhmrc/publications/attachments/cd33_infection_control_healthcare.pdf.
8. Australian Commission on Safety and Quality in Health Care, *Safety and Quality Improvement Guide Standard 3: Preventing and Controlling Healthcare Associated Infections* (2012), available at: http://www.safetyandquality.gov.au/publications/safety-and-quality-improvement-guide-standard-3-preventing-and-controlling-healthcare-associated-infections-october-2012/; M.D. Valim, M.H. Palucci Marziale, M. Richart-Martinez and A. Sanjuan-Quiles, 'Instruments for Evaluating Compliance with Infection Control Practices and Factors That Affect It: An Integrative Review,' *Journal of Clinical Nursing* 23 (2014): 1502–19.

9. T.B. Rogers, N.A. Kuiper and W.S. Kirker, 'Self-Reference and the Encoding of Personal Information,' *Journal of Personality and Social Psychology* 35 (1997): 677–88.
10. V. O'Donnell, *Television Criticism* (Los Angeles, CA: Sage, 2007).
11. S. Pokornowski, 'Insecure Lives: Zombies, Global Health, and the Totalitarianism of Generalization,' *Literature and Medicine* 31 (2014): 216–34.
12. C. Foreman, 'Witchcraft Science in the Cinema of Epidemics,' *Science Communication* 17 (1995): 3–8.
13. M. Johnson, 'More than Pop Culture: Depictions of HIV in the Media and the Effect on Viewer's Perception of Risk,' *Journal of Homosexuality* 60, no. 8 (2013): 1117–42.
14. J. McCullough, *Zombies: A Hunter's Guide* (Oxford: Osprey Publishing, 2010).
15. M. Brooks, *The Zombie Survival Guide. Complete Protection from the Living Dead* (New York: Three Rivers Press, 2003); P. Munz, I. Hudea, J. Imad and T. Smith, 'When Zombies Attack!: Mathematical Modelling of an Outbreak of Zombie Infection,' in *Infectious Disease Modelling Research Progress*, ed. J. Tchuenche and C. Chiyaka (New York: Nova Science Publishers, 2009), 133–50; M. Montandon, *The Proper Care and Feeding of Zombies: A Completely Scientific Guide to the Lives of the Un-Dead* (Hoboken, NJ: John Wiley & Sons, 2010).
16. Wikipedia, 'List of Zombie Films' (2014), available at: http://en.wikipedia.org/wiki/List_of_zombie_films.
17. Ibid.
18. World Health Organization, *Disease Outbreaks by Year* (2014), available at: http://www.who.int/csr/don/archive/year/en/.
19. K. Bishop, 'Dead Man Still Walking: Explaining the Zombie Renaissance,' *Journal of Popular Film and Television* 37 (2009): 16–25.
20. A. Lane, 'Personal Communication. Producer/Director "Invasion of the Not Quite Dead",' London, 2014.
21. Centers for Disease Control and Prevention, 'Zombie Preparedness' (2014), available at: http://www.cdc.gov/phpr/zombies.html.
22. United States Strategic Command, 'CDR SSTRATCOM CO~PLAN 8888-Ll 'COUNTER-ZOMBIE DOMINANCE' 30 APR 2011' (2014), available at: http://www.stratcom.mil/files/foia_requests/CONPLAN8888-11.pdf.
23. P. Munz et al., 'When Zombies Attack!'; M. Nasiruddin, M. Halabi, A. Dao, K. Chen and B. Brown, 'Zombies—A Pop Culture Resource for Public Health Awareness,' *Emerging Infectious Diseases* 19 (2013): 809–13; J. Verran, M. Crossley, K. Carolan, N. Jacobs and M. Amos, 'Monsters, Microbiology and Mathematics: The Epidemiology of a

Zombie Apocalypse,' *Journal of Biological Education* 48, no. 2 (2014): 98–104.

24. Traffic Accident Commission, 'TAC 20 Year Anniversary Retrospective Montage "Everybody Hurts"' (2015), available at: https://www.tac.vic. gov.au/road-safety/tac-campaigns/20-year-campaign.
25. A. Mattu, 'Lessons from the Princess Bride' (2015), available at: http:// www.smacc.net.au/2015/10/lessons-from-the-princess-bride/.
26. E. Wright, *Shaun of the Dead* (England: Universal Pictures, 2004); D. Boyle, *28 Days Later*, (England: DNA Films, 2002).
27. Wright, *Shaun of the Dead*; M. Spierig and P. Spierig, *Undead*, (Australia: Spierig Film, 2003).
28. D. Stanley, 'The Nurses' Role in the Prevention of Solanum Infection: Dealing with a Zombie Epidemic,' *Journal of Clinical Nursing* 21, nos. 11–12 (2012): 1606–13.
29. Ibid.
30. L.D. Lowe and F.I. Hummel, 'Disaster Readiness for Nurses in the Workplace: Preparing for the Zombie Apocalypse,' *Workplace Health & Safety* 62, no. 5 (2014): 207–13; Centers for Disease Control and Prevention 'Zombie Preparedness.'
31. P. Chamings, 'Is it Professionally Acceptable for a Nurse to Stay Home during a Pandemic? 2nd Opinion: Writing for the Pro Position,' *The American Journal of Maternal/Child Nursing* 33 (2008): 202–3. Lowe and Hummel, 'Disaster Readiness for Nurses in the Workplace.'
32. Brooks, The Zombie Survival Guide.
33. Ibid.; Peta-Anne Zimmerman, Matt Mason and Elizabeth Elder, 'A Healthy Degree of Suspicion: A Discussion of the Implementation of Transmission Based Precautions in the Emergency Department,' *Australasian Emergency Nursing Journal* 19, no. 3 (2016): 149–52.
34. N. Cassir, S. Boudjema, V. Roux, P. Brouqui, P. Reynier and T. No. 'Infectious Diseases of High Consequence and Personal Protective Equipment: A Didactic Method to Assess the Risk of Contamination. Infection Control & Hospital Epidemiology.' *Infection Control and Hospital Epidemiology* 36, no. 12 (2015): doi: 10.1017/ice.2015.223; M. Tomas, S. Kundrapu, P. Thota et al. 'Contamination of Health Care Personnel During Removal of Personal Protective Equipment,' *JAMA Intern Medicine* 175, no. 12 (2015): 1904–10.

## BIBLIOGRAPHY

Allen, J.A., J. Currey and J. Considine, 'Annual Resuscitation Competency Assessments: A Review of the Evidence,' *Australian Critical Care: Official Journal of the Confederation of Australian Critical Care Nurses* 26, no. 1 (2013): 12–7.

Australian Commission on Safety and Quality in Health Care. 'Safety and Quality Improvement Guide Standard 3: Preventing and Controlling Healthcare Associated Infections' (2012), available at: http://www.safetyandquality.gov.au/publications/safety-and-quality-improvement-guide-standard-3-preventing-and-controlling-healthcare-associated-infections-october-2012/.

Bishop, K. 'Dead Man Still Walking: Explaining the Zombie Renaissance.' *Journal of Popular Film and Television* 37 (2009): 16–25.

Boon, Kevin Alexander. 'Ontological Anxiety Made Flesh: The Zombie in Literature, Film and Culture.' In *Monsters and the Monstrous:Myths and Metaphors of Enduring Evil,* ed. Niall Scott. Amsterdam: Rodopi, 2007, 33–44.

Boyle, D. *28 Days Later.* England: DNA Films, 2002.

Brooks, M. *The Zombie Survival Guide. Complete Protection from the Living Dead.* New York: Three Rivers Press, 2003.

Cassir, N., S. Boudjema, V. Roux, P. Brouqui, P. Reynier and T. No, 'Infectious Diseases of High Consequence and Personal Protective Equipment: A Didactic Method to Assess the Risk of Contamination. Infection Control & Hospital Epidemiology.' *Infection Control and Hospital Epidemiology* 36, no. 12 (2015): doi: 10.1017/ice.2015.223.

Centers for Disease Control and Prevention. *Zombie Preparedness* (2014), available at: http://www.cdc.gov/phpr/zombies.html.

Chamings, P. 'Is It Professionally Acceptable for a Nurse to Stay Home during a Pandemic? 2nd Opinion: Writing for the Pro Position.' *The American Journal of Maternal/Child Nursing* 33 (2008): 202–3.

Clinical Excellence Commission. 'Healthcare Associated Infections Program' (2015), available at: http://www.cec.health.nsw.gov.au/programs/hai.

Foreman, C. 'Witchcraft Science in the Cinema of Epidemics.' *Science Communication* 17 (1995): 3–8.

'History of Zombies.' 2016. http://anthropology.msu.edu/anp264-ss13/2013/04/25/history-of-zombies/.

Jenkins, H., R. Purushotma, M. Weigel, K. Clinton and A.J. Robinson, *Confronting the Challenges of Participatory Culture: Media Education for the 21st Century.* Cambridge, MA: MIT Press, 2009.

Johnson, M. 'More than Pop Culture: Depictions of HIV in the Media and the Effect on Viewer's Perception of Risk,' *Journal of Homosexuality* 60, no. 8 (2013): 1117–42.

Kline, Jim. 'Zombie Typology.' *Psychological Perspectives* 55 (2012): 467–81.

Lane, A. 'Personal Communication. Producer/Director "Invasion of the Not Quite Dead".' London, 2014.

Lowe, L.D. and F.I. Hummel, 'Disaster Readiness for Nurses in the Workplace: Preparing for the Zombie Apocalypse,' *Workplace Health & Safety* 62, no. 5 (2014): 207–13.

Mattu, A. 'Lessons from the Princess Bride' (2015), available at: http://www.smacc.net.au/2015/10/lessons-from-the-princess-bride/.

McCullough, J. *Zombies: A Hunter's Guide.* Oxford: Osprey Publishing, 2010.

Montandon, M. *The Proper Care and Feeding of Zombies: A Completely Scientific Guide to the Lives of the Un-Dead.* Hoboken, NJ: John Wiley & Sons, 2010.

Nasiruddin, M., M. Halabi, A. Dao, K. Chen and B. Brown, 'Zombies—A Pop Culture Resource for Public Health Awareness,' *Emerging Infectious Diseases* 19 (2013): 809–13.

National Health and Medical Research Council. *Australian Guidelines for the Prevention and Control of Infection in Healthcare.* Canberra: Commonwealth of Australia (2010), available at: http://www.legislationreview.nhmrc.gov.au/_files_nhmrc/publications/attachments/cd33_infection_control_health-care.pdf.

O'Donnell, V. *Television Criticism.* Los Angeles, CA: Sage, 2007.

Pokornowski, S. 'Insecure Lives: Zombies, Global Health, and the Totalitarianism of Generalization.' *Literature and Medicine* 31 (2014): 216–34.

Rogers, T.B., N.A. Kuiper and W.S. Kirker, 'Self-Reference and the Encoding of Personal Information.' *Journal of Personality and Social Psychology* 35 (1977): 677–88.

Spierig, M. and P. Spierig, *Undead.* Australia: Spierig Film, 2003.

Stanley, D. 'The Nurses' Role in the Prevention of Solanum Infection: Dealing with a Zombie Epidemic.' *Journal of Clinical Nursing* 21, nos. 11–12 (2012): 1606–13.

Tchuenche, J. and C. Chiyaka, eds. *Infectious Disease Modelling Research Progress.* New York: Nova Science Publishers, 2009.

Tomas, M, S. Kundrapu, P. Thota et al. 'Contamination of Health Care Personnel During Removal of Personal Protective Equipment,' *JAMA Intern Medicine* 175, no. 12 (2015): 1904–10.

Traffic Accident Commission. 'TAC 20 Year Anniversary Retrospective Montage "Everybody Hurts"' (2015), available at: https://www.tac.vic.gov.au/road-safety/tac-campaigns/20-year-campaign.

United States Strategic Command. 'CDR SSTRATCOM CO~PLAN 8888-Ll 'COUNTER-ZOMBIE DOMINANCE' 30 APR 2011' (2014), available at: http://www.stratcom.mil/files/foia_requests/CONPLAN8888-11.pdf.

Valim, M.D., M.H. Palucci Marziale, M. Richart-Martinez and A. Sanjuan-Quiles, 'Instruments for Evaluating Compliance with Infection Control Practices and Factors That Affect It: An Integrative Review.' *Journal of Clinical Nursing* 23 (2014): 1502–19.

Verran, J., M. Crossley, K. Carolan, N. Jacobs and M. Amos, 'Monsters, Microbiology and Mathematics: The Epidemiology of a Zombie Apocalypse.' *Journal of Biological Education* 48, no. 2 (2014): 98–104.

Wikipedia. 'List of Zombie Films' (2014), available at: http://en.wikipedia.org/wiki/List_of_Zombie_films.

World Health Organization, *Disease Outbreaks by Year* (2014), available at: http://www.who.int/csr/don/archive/year/en/.

———. *WHO: Clean Care Is Safer Care* (2015), available at: http://www.who.int/gpsc/en/.

Wright, E. *Shaun of the Dead*. England: Universal Pictures, 2004.

Zimmerman, Peta-Anne, Matt Mason and Elizabeth Elder. 'A Healthy Degree of Suspicion: A Discussion of the Implementation of Transmission Based Precautions in the Emergency Department.' *Australasian Emergency Nursing Journal* 19, no. 3 (2016): 149–52.

## CHAPTER 5

# Celebrity? Doctor? Celebrity Doctor? Which Spokesperson is Most Effective for Cancer Prevention?

*Candice-Brooke Woods, Stacey Baxter, Elizabeth King, Kerrin Palazzi, Christopher Oldmeadow and Erica L. James*

C.-B. Woods (✉) · E.L. James · S. Baxter
University of Newcastle, Callaghan, NSW, Australia
e-mail: Candice.Woods@uon.edu.au

E.L. James
e-mail: Erica.James@newcastle.edu.au

S. Baxter
e-mail: Stacey.Baxter@newcastle.edu.au

E. King
Cancer Council NSW, Woolloomooloo, NSW, Australia
e-mail: Elizabeth.King@nswcc.org.au

K. Palazzi · C. Oldmeadow
Clinical Research Design, Information and Statistical Support, Hunter
Medical Research Institute, New Lambton Heights, NSW, Australia
e-mail: Kerrin.Palazzi@hmri.org.au

C. Oldmeadow
e-mail: Christopher.Oldmeadow@hmri.org.au

© The Author(s) 2017                                                        71
E. Kendal and B. Diug (eds.), *Teaching Medicine and Medical Ethics
Using Popular Culture*, Palgrave Studies in Science and Popular Culture,
DOI 10.1007/978-3-319-65451-5_5

The use of celebrity spokespersons in advertising is well established in commercial marketing.[1] Celebrities who are considered attractive and familiar to target audiences have been shown to lead to positive attitudes toward the brand, advertisement and increased purchase intentions.[2] Subsequently, celebrities are increasingly being utilised in the not-for-profit (NFP) sector, specifically as part of social marketing campaigns.[3] NFP organisations often utilise well-known and recognised celebrities based on their ability to influence fundraising efforts, draw attention to social causes and potentially influence those with political power.[4]

The selection of an appropriate spokesperson enhances message tangibility, and is considered an important part of strategic message development.[5] The character and credibility of a spokesperson can significantly impact the persuasiveness of an advertisement's message.[6] The credibility of the spokesperson (referred to in the marketing literature as source credibility) is traditionally operationalised via three dimensions: expertise, trustworthiness and attractiveness.[7] Whilst the influence of source credibility (and its separate dimensions) has been explored for different spokesperson types within a commercial marketing context, there is much less research in the overall NFP social marketing context.[8] Health behaviour change theory recommends that an emphasis should be placed on the expertise of the spokesperson.[9] Furthermore, it is suggested that health-related decision-making may differ from that of general consumer decisions, with public health advertising designed to promote voluntary changes in health behaviours and the cessation of unhealthy behaviours rather than attempting to influence purchasing behaviours.[10]

This chapter investigates the effects that spokesperson type (celebrity, medical doctor, celebrity doctor) and source characteristics (expertise versus familiarity) have on an individual's intention to act on health-based social marketing messages.

## LITERATURE REVIEW

Public Service Announcements (PSAs) are a valuable tool used in developing public health mass media campaigns that target health behaviour change.[11] Cancer-related PSAs are commonly utilised by government, charitable and non-profit cancer organisations to raise awareness, educate about signs and symptoms of different cancers, promote available screening methods and address risk behaviours.[12] To deliver these messages, a spokesperson is often engaged as part of public health mass media campaigns. For example, Public Health England (PHE), in partnership with the Department of Health, NHS England and Cancer Research UK, has involved a variety of spokesperson types for the 'Be Clear on Cancer' campaigns which target lung cancer prevention; from public support and involvement from well-known figures, such as comedian Ricky Gervais (2012), to real medical doctors (2016), promoting the health message 'tell your doctor' if experiencing signs and symptoms.[13]

Within health-based messages, such as the PHE example above, a medical doctor is employed as an *expert spokesperson*;[14] academically qualified and with a large emphasis placed on their profession. A professional expert spokesperson is defined as 'a recognized authority on the product class endorsed whose expertise, the result of special knowledge or training, is superior to that acquired by ordinary people.'[15] Medical doctors are commonly cast within advertisements as qualification-based professional experts, for example, featuring as health authorities in pharmaceutical commercials.[16] Medical doctors have a trusted and respected image within the community.[17] For example, a 2016 research survey (United Kingdom) showed 'Doctors' to be the most trusted profession, with '89% of the public trusting them to tell the truth.'[18]

It is expected that a spokesperson recognised by audiences as being a professional medical expert will enhance the effectiveness of a PSA health message. Previous research has identified expertise as being a key factor for a spokesperson to inhabit to effectively persuade audience attitudes, opinions and create behaviour change, and has been suggested as being the most important dimension of source credibility.[19] Expert endorsements have the ability to enhance message strength, believability and compliance, primarily owing to credibility.[20] Spokespersons perceived as having high expertise, experience and status also encourage greater levels of judgement and imitative behaviours.[21] Several studies have shown a positive association between the expertise of a spokesperson, attitude and behavioural change.[22] There are few studies, however, which investigate the effectiveness of medical doctors as health spokespersons. Hu and Sundar (2009) compared the online environment influence of doctors versus laypersons on perceived credibility and behavioural intention, results confirming that participants generally favoured 'the expertise of medical professionals over laypersons except in the case of blog and Internet as a whole.'[23] Braunsberger and Munch (1998) showed that doctors are more persuasive than unknown spokespersons, who were perceived to be low in expertise.[24]

A *celebrity*, on the other hand, is often engaged as an attractive, familiar source; well known and recognisable by audiences for their achievements in an area unrelated to the advertisement, with a perceived personal interest in the campaign.[25] A celebrity spokesperson is defined as 'an individual who is known by the public (actor, sports figure, entertainer, etc.) for his or her achievements in areas other than that of the product class endorsed.'[26] In a commercial marketing context, celebrities are commonly selected as product spokespersons for their abilities to generate media coverage, achieve high recall, capacity to increase brand visibility and familiarity with target audiences, as well as being able to persuade behavioural changes.[27] An extensive body of literature supports celebrity-based advertising,[28] presenting celebrity spokespersons as effective in the dimensions of trustworthiness, believability, persuasiveness and likeability,[29] as well as acting as a peripheral heuristic cue for consumers less involved with an advertisement message.[30]

It is expected that a celebrity who is familiar to target audiences will influence the effectiveness of a PSA health message. Familiarity is an important characteristic for marketing doctors to consider when selecting a celebrity spokesperson.[31] Research indicates that familiar spokespersons are perceived as being more attractive, knowledgeable and identifiable,[32] as well as enhancing endorser effectiveness.[33] Many health-related PSAs featuring celebrities have been linked with effectively encouraging intention and behaviour change in both adults and youth.[34]

A third potential spokesperson type is the celebrity doctor (for example, Dr. Mehmet Oz, *The Dr. Oz Show*). Celebrity doctors have been reported as having significant influence over television ratings and audience persuasion.[35]

In summary, further investigation is required for research that directly compares the effectiveness of medical doctors and celebrities as spokespersons for health-related PSAs. Based on the above evidence, and the health-based nature of the PSA, we expect that a medical doctor will be perceived as having a higher level of source expertise than a celebrity health spokesperson, and anticipate that the association, at least in part, between health spokesperson and participant behavioural intentions may be mediated through expertise. We expect a celebrity spokesperson to be rated as more familiar to participants than a medical doctor, and that behavioural intention will be influenced as an indirect result of public knowledge and familiarity of the spokesperson. Both medical doctors and celebrity doctors have relevant expertise, but we anticipate that the perceived expertise of a celebrity doctor will be heightened through public familiarity. Skin cancer prevention in Australia is used as the public health PSA scenario for this study.

Finally, it is important to consider audience preferences. Health practitioners are increasingly being encouraged to support the wants and needs of the patient, considering among other things patient preferences in treatment decision-making, and to recognise the differences that exist between the judgement of health professionals and patients' knowledge of their own health.[36] Health information tailored to meet audience needs can assist with increasing health literacy and in 'reinforcing professionals' explanations of health problems.'[37] We argue that it is important to consider the preference of the PSA audience into health campaign advertising decisions. Based on the evidence above, we expect participants to report a higher preference for a medical doctor over a celebrity.

## METHOD

### *Aim*

Part one of this study aims to compare a celebrity and medical doctor as health spokespersons on behavioural intention for skin cancer prevention print advertising. More specifically, we examine whether the association between health spokesperson (medical doctor versus celebrity) and participant behavioural intentions is mediated through the perceived source expertise and familiarity of the spokesperson. Part two compares a medical doctor (expert) and a celebrity doctor (familiar expert) on behavioural intention for skin cancer prevention, and to assess the mediating role of familiarity and expertise.

### *Participants*

Eligibility for both studies was restricted to participants aged 14–80 years, who were fluent in English and who had internet access. Participants were recruited using quota sampling from a nationwide registered research panel.[38] Sample size calculations to attain a statistical power of 0.80, with an effect size $f = 0.25$ and a priori $\alpha = 0.05$ were achieved, with a sample of 224 for study one and 225 for study two.[39]

## Design

Two separate randomised between-subjects studies were performed, allocating participants to one of two experimental conditions, followed by an online survey. Participants were presented with a mock print Cancer Council NSW advertisement, displaying the image of either a celebrity or generic medical doctor (Part one), or a generic medical doctor or celebrity doctor (Part two); the only notable difference between advertisements being the health spokesperson image used. After collection of demographics, participants were asked to rate the expertise and familiarity of the spokesperson, their intention to act on the messages provided, and who they would prefer to receive health advice from.

### Measures

Expertise was measured using five questions and a seven-point semantic differential scale: *Not an expert/an expert, inexperienced/experienced, unknowledgeable/knowledgeable, unqualified/qualified* and *unskilled/skilled*.[40] Familiarity of the spokesperson was assessed using two seven-point semantic differential scales: *not very familiar/very familiar,* and *don't know very well/know very well*.[41] Participant behavioural intention was measured,[42] using three seven-point semantic differential scales: *unlikely/likely, definitely not/definitely* and *improbably/probably*. Cronbach's alpha was used to test internal consistancy for the expertise, familiarity and intention questions; mean scores were then computed by averaging the questions. Finally, participants were asked to report who they would prefer to receive health advice from, across three options: *Celebrity, Medical Doctor* or *Celebrity Doctor*.

### Mock Print PSA Stimuli Development

Pre-testing followed procedures employed by Ohanian (1990) with a sample ($n = 36$) of university students recalling celebrity names, a second group ($n = 36$) rating the celebrities on *familiarity* and *attitude*.[43] Taylor Swift was selected as the celebrity used in study one ($M_{familiarity} = 5.9$   $SD = 1.4$,   $p < 0.001$;   $M_{Attitudes} = 4.8$,   $SD = 1.8$, $p = 0.013$; name recall $= 94.4\%$). The medical doctor counterpart for Taylor Swift was chosen from *iStock by Getty Images* (istockphoto.com) to reflect the age and appearance of the celebrity,[44] and a final group

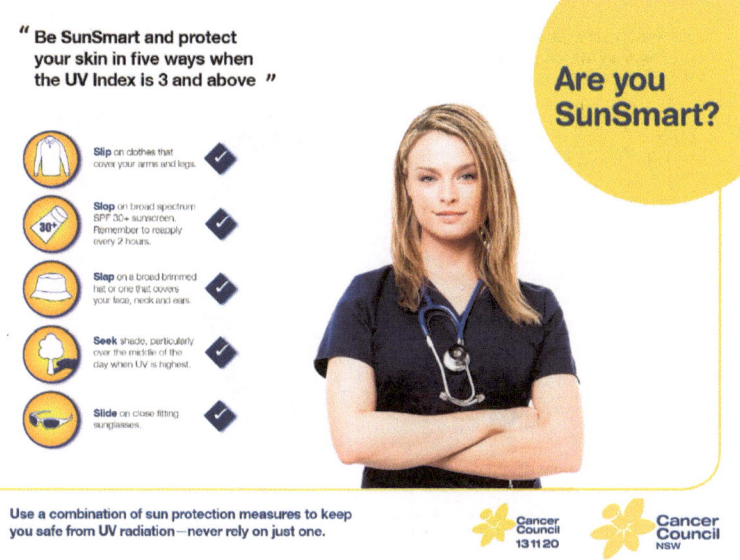

**Fig. 5.1** Example mock print PSA stimuli—medical doctor (study one) (*Mock print PSA stimuli for this study were created by adapting an original resource developed by the Cancer Council South Australia, and use of the Program name 'SunSmart' developed by the Cancer Council Victoria. Spokesperson images sourced from iStock by Getty Images.*)

of university students ($n = 40$) assessed the degree of physical similarity between the celebrity and chosen medical doctor stimuli.[45] Dr. Oz was selected as the celebrity doctor stimulus, receiving the highest named frequency from a list of celebrity doctors identified during pretest ($n = 27$). The generic male medical doctor was also selected from istockphoto.com. The mock print PSAs for this study were created by adapting an original resource developed by the Cancer Council South Australia, and use of the program name '*SunSmart*' developed by the Cancer Council Victoria[46] (Figs. 5.1 and 5.2).

## Analysis

Crude (unadjusted) expertise (and its five comprising components), familiarity, and intention scores are presented as mean (standard

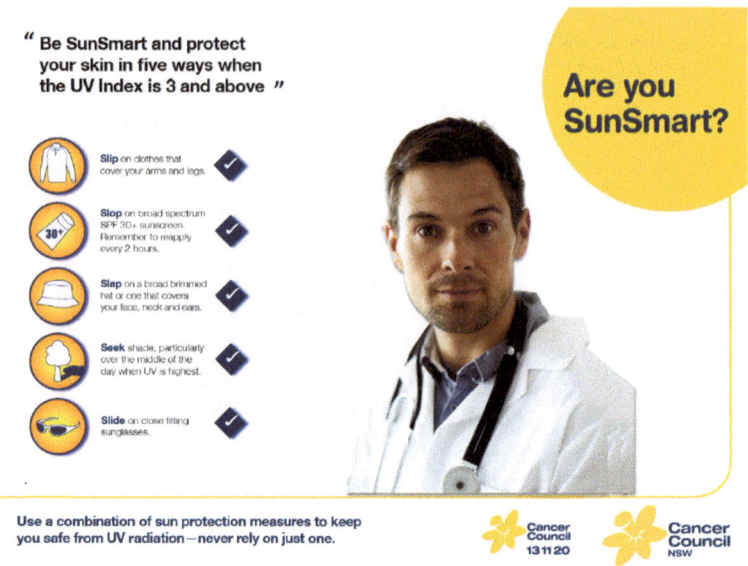

**Fig. 5.2**  Example mock print PSA stimuli—medical doctor (study two) (*Mock print PSA stimuli for this study were created by adapting an original resource developed by the Cancer Council South Australia, and use of the Program name 'SunSmart' developed by the Cancer Council Victoria. Spokesperson images sourced from iStock by Getty Images.*)

deviation; SD), and were compared between the two spokesperson types using independent samples t-test. Participant preferred choice of health spokesperson is presented as count (%) and compared between spokesperson types using Pearson Chi-squared test. To further examine the hypothesised relationships, mediation analysis was performed according to the methods of Preacher & Hayes (2004) using structural equation modelling. Mediation through both expertise and familiarity was examined within one model (dual mediation); estimates (β) presented include the mean difference in intention between the two spokesperson types (i.e. the total effect), estimates of the effects attributable to being mediated through expertise or familiarity (indirect effects), and an estimate of the effect that is not through these mediators (direct effect). These estimates are presented with 95% confidence intervals (CI) and p-values obtained from bootstrapping (n = 1000 bootstrapped samples).

Additionally, $p$-values are presented for the test of equality of the indirect pathways for the two mediators.

## RESULTS

### Study One: Celebrity Versus Medical Doctor

In total, 224 participants (male $= 123$, $M_{age} = 45$, $SD = 20.6$) participated in study one. Internal consistency was measured and found to be high for expertise ($\alpha = 0.948$), familiarity ($\alpha = 0.968$) and intention ($\alpha = 0.977$). There was no difference between a celebrity and a medical doctor in participant intention to act on cancer preventative messages (crude $M_{Medical\ Doctor\ Intention} = 4.9$, $SD = 1.6$; $M_{Celebrity\ Intention} = 4.7$, $SD = 1.8$, $p = 0.406$) (Table 5.1). However, as hypothesised, participants perceived a medical doctor as having a higher level of expertise than a celebrity spokesperson (crude $M_{Medical\ Doctor} = 5.03$, $SD = 1.2$; $M_{Celebrity} = 4.4$, $SD = 1.4$; $p < 0.001$). This was also found for each of the five individual components of source expertise. After adjusting for familiarity, higher source expertise was also found to be associated with higher behavioural intention to follow cancer preventative PSA messages ($\beta = 0.5$, $p < 0.001$; Table 5.2). A significant indirect effect was observed for health spokesperson type on participant intention to act through source expertise ($\beta = -0.3$, $p = 0.002$). Moreover, as hypothesised, participants perceived a celebrity as having higher levels of familiarity than the medical doctor (crude $M_{Medical\ Doctor} = 2.7$, $SD = 1.8$; $M_{Celebrity} = 4.3$, $SD = 2.02$; $p < 0.001$); however, after adjusting for expertise, higher familiarity scores were not statistically significantly

**Table 5.1** Health spokesperson effects (part one): Summary of crude means (SD)

|  | Medical doctor | Celebrity | p-Value |
|---|---|---|---|
| Intention | 4.9 (1.6) | 4.7 (1.7) | 0.409 |
| Familiarity | 2.7 (1.76) | 4.3 (2.0) | <0.001* |
| Expertise | 5.03 (1.2) | 4.4 (1.4) | 0.001* |
| – *An expert* | 4.79 (1.3) | 4.03 (1.7) | <0.001* |
| – *Experienced* | 4.99 (1.28) | 4.5 (1.5) | 0.015* |
| – *Knowledgeable* | 5.17 (1.3) | 4.7 (1.6) | 0.014* |
| – *Qualified* | 5.1 (1.3) | 4.3 (1.6) | <0.001* |
| – *Skilled* | 5.08 (1.3) | 4.62 (1.5) | 0.014* |

*Significant at $p < 0.05$ using independent t-test

**Table 5.2** Mediating effects of health spokesperson expertise and familiarity on behavioural intention (part one)

|  | β | 95% CI | p-Value |
|---|---|---|---|
| **Effect 1a**: Association of spokesperson on familiarity | 1.5 | 1.04, 2.03 | <0.001* |
| **Effect 1b:** Association of familiarity on intention | 0.7 | −0.04, 0.18 | 0.219 |
| **Indirect effect (1a*1b)** of spokesperson on intention, through familiarity | 0.1 | −0.07, 0.28 | 0.233 |
| **Effect 2a**: Association of spokesperson on expertise | −0.6 | −0.94, −0.26 | 0.001* |
| **Effect 2b:** Association of expertise on intention | 0.5 | 0.35, 0.66 | <0.001* |
| **Indirect effect (2a*2b)** of spokesperson on intention, through expertise | −0.3 | −0.5, −0.11 | 0.002* |
| **Total effect** of spokesperson on intention (without mediators) | −0.19 | −0.63, 0.25 | 0.406 |
| **Direct effect** of spokesperson on intention (with mediators) | 0.01 | −0.44, 0.46 | 0.967 |

*Significant at $p < 0.05$ using structural equation modelling
β = beta coefficient

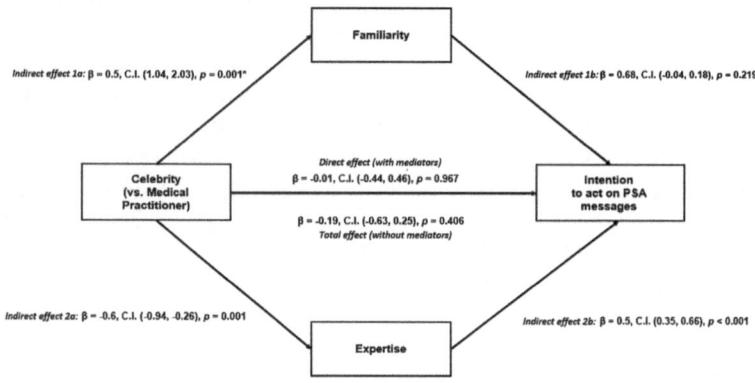

**Fig. 5.3** Mediation analysis: Celebrity versus medical doctor (part one)

associated with higher behavioural intention ($\beta = 0.07$, $p = 0.219$). After adjusting for mediation through expertise and familiarity, no statistically significant direct effect was observed between the health spokesperson and behavioural intention ($\beta = 0.01$, $p = 0.967$; see Fig. 5.3). Overall, 92% ($n = 206$) of respondents reported that they would prefer information from a medical doctor; rather than a celebrity (3.6%) or a

**Table 5.3** Participant spokesperson preference (count % within participant group) (part one)

| | Health Spokesperson PSA Group (count % within participant group) | | Total (%) |
| --- | --- | --- | --- |
| | Medical Doctor (%) | Celebrity (%) | |
| Celebrity | 2 (1.8) | 6 (5.3) | 8 (3.6) |
| Medical Doctor | 106 (95.5) | 100 (88.5) | 206 (92.0) |
| Celebrity Doctor | 3 (2.7) | 7 (6.2) | 10 (4.5) |
| Total | 111 (100) | 113 (100) | 224 (100) |

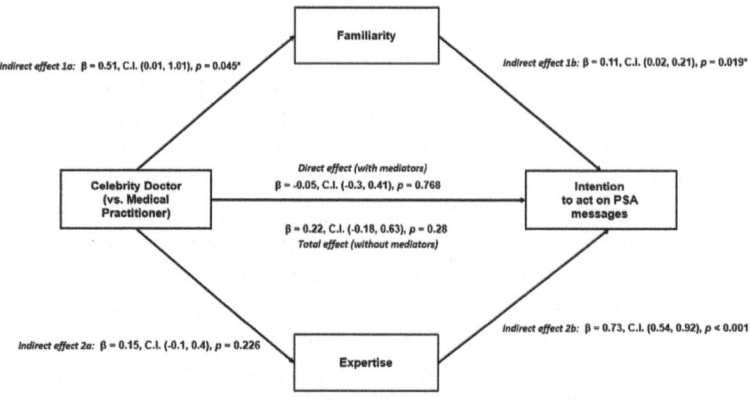

**Fig. 5.4** Mediation analysis: Celebrity doctor versus medical doctor (part two)

celebrity doctor (4.5%; Table 5.3). Spokesperson preference for information from a medical professional was not significantly different between celebrity and medical doctor groups (88.5% vs. 95.5% respectively; $p = 0.153$) (Fig. 5.4).

### Study Two: Medical Doctor Versus Celebrity Doctor

A separate sample of 225 members of the Australian public (117 male, 106 female, two transgender/intersex/unidentified, $M_{age} = 45$, range 14–79 years, $SD = 20.6$) participated in part two of this study. Both the celebrity doctor and medical doctor were equally effective at directly

**Table 5.4**  Health spokesperson effects (part one): Summary of crude means (SD)

|  | Medical Doctor | Celebrity Doctor | p-Value |
|---|---|---|---|
| Intention | 5.0 (1.5) | 5.2 (1.6) | 0.637 |
| Familiarity | 2.5 (1.9) | 3.04 (2.0) | 0.048* |
| Expertise | 4.7 (0.9) | 4.9 (1.0) | 0.229 |
| – An expert | 4.8 (1.5) | 5.2 (1.2) | 0.029 |
| – Experienced | 4.84 (1.4) | 5.2 (1.2) | 0.071 |
| – Knowledgeable | 5.03 (1.3) | 5.3 (1.2) | 0.136 |
| – Qualified | 5.03 (1.5) | 5.3 (1.2) | 0.143 |
| – Skilled | 5.02 (1.5) | 5.2 (1.2) | 0.282 |

*Significant at $p < 0.05$ using independent t-test

impacting participant intention to act on cancer preventative messages (crude $M_{\text{Medical Doctor Intention}} = 5.0$, $SD = 1.5$; $M_{\text{Celebrity Doctor Intention}} = 5.2$, $SD = 1.6$; $p = 0.28$) (Table 5.4). No significant difference was found between the spokesperson type and source expertise (crude $M_{\text{Medical Doctor Expertise}} = 4.7$, $SD = 0.9$; $M_{\text{Celebrity Doctor Expertise}} = 4.9$, $SD = 1.0$; $p = 0.229$), suggesting that participants perceived a celebrity doctor as being equal in medical expertise to a medical doctor spokesperson. This was also found for four of the five scale individual components of source expertise. Adjusting for familiarity, higher source expertise was found to be associated with higher behavioural intention to follow cancer preventative PSA messages ($\beta = 0.73$, $p < 0.001$; see Table 5.5). Overall, no statistically significant indirect effect was observed for health spokesperson type on participant intention to act through source expertise ($\beta = 0.11$, $p = 0.233$). Participants perceived a celebrity doctor as having higher levels of familiarity (crude $M_{\text{Medical Doctor}} = 2.5$, $SD = 1.9$; $M_{\text{Celebrity Dr}} = 3.04$, $SD = 2.0$; $p = 0.048$). After adjusting for expertise, higher familiarity scores were also found associated with higher behavioural intention ($\beta = 0.11$, $p = 0.019$); however, no significant indirect effect was observed between the health spokesperson and behavioural intention through familiarity ($\beta = 0.06$, $p = 0.120$). Overall, 93.8% ($n = 211$) of respondents reported that they would prefer information from a medical doctor; rather than a celebrity (2.7%) or a celebrity doctor (3.6%; see Table 5.6). Spokesperson preference was not significantly different between celebrity and medical doctor groups (93.6% versus 93.9% respectively; $p = 0.556$).

**Table 5.5**  Mediating effects of health spokesperson expertise and familiarity on behavioural intention (part two)

| | $\beta$ | 95% CI | p-Value |
|---|---|---|---|
| **Effect 1a:** Association of spokesperson on familiarity | 0.51 | 0.01, 1.01 | 0.045* |
| **Effect 1b:** Association of familiarity on intention | 0.11 | 0.02, 0.21 | 0.019* |
| **Indirect effect (1a\*1b)** of spokesperson on intention, through familiarity | 0.06 | −0.02, 0.13 | 0.120 |
| **Effect 2a:** Association of spokesperson on expertise | 0.15 | −0.1, 0.4 | 0.226 |
| **Effect 2b:** Association of expertise on intention | 0.73 | 0.54, 0.92 | <0.001* |
| **Indirect effect (2a\*2b)** of spokesperson on intention, through expertise | 0.11 | −0.07, 0.3 | 0.233 |
| **Total effect** of spokesperson on intention (without mediators) | 0.22 | −0.18, 0.63 | 0.28 |
| **Direct effect** of spokesperson on intention (with mediators) | 0.05 | −0.3, 0.41 | 0.768 |

*Significant at $p < 0.05$ using structural equation modelling
$\beta$ = beta coefficient

**Table 5.6**  Participant spokesperson preference (count % within participant group) (part two)

| | Health Spokesperson PSA Group (count % within participant group) | | Total (%) |
|---|---|---|---|
| | Medical Doctor (%) | Celebrity Doctor (%) | |
| Celebrity | 4 (3.6) | 2 (1.7) | 6 (2.7) |
| Medical Doctor | 103 (93.6) | 108 (93.9) | 211 (93.8) |
| Celebrity Doctor | 3 (2.7) | 5 (4.3) | 8 (3.6) |
| Total | 110 (100) | 115 (100) | 225 (100) |

### Discussion and Conclusion

There were no statistically significant differences between a celebrity and medical doctor influencing audience intention to follow advertised health advice. Important differences were noted, however, for the expertise and familiarity scores for the health spokesperson types. After adjusting for familiarity, a significant association was found for audience intention to act on health advertising messages through source. Though the celebrity health spokesperson had higher familiarity amongst participants, after adjusting for expertise, this did not translate into increased behavioural intention, rejecting our anticipated hypothesis that celebrity familiarity would increase participant intention to act on health PSA messages. Further, participants overwhelmingly reported a preference for receipt of health information from a medical doctor rather than a celebrity.

Similarly, there was also no statistically significant difference between a medical doctor and celebrity doctor on audience intention to follow advertised health advice. No significant differences were found between the two health spokesperson types for source expertise, demonstrating a shared audience perception that a celebrity doctor and medical doctor have similar medical expertise when presenting cancer prevention messages. As expected, after adjusting for source expertise, participants reported higher familiarity with a celebrity doctor. While familiarity was found to have a significant positive influence on participant behavioural intentions, consistent with study one, no significant association was found for audience intention to act on health advertising messages through spokesperson familiarity.

Though familiarity of a spokesperson is important, the findings of this study emphasise the importance of perceived expertise in health-based advertising. Drawing from source credibility theory, *expertise* is recognised as a level of experience, skill, 'valid assertions' or knowledge held by a spokesperson.[47] When a message is delivered from a highly credible source, consumers are more likely to be persuaded and accept an advertisement's arguments.[48] Findings from this study complement previous research of medical doctors being recognised as a source of expertise,[49] and also support the positive influence source expertise has on effectively persuading behaviour change.[50]

## IMPLICATIONS

These findings have implications for those planning cancer prevention social marketing campaigns. Since the nature and subject of preventative cancer advertisements are medically orientated, the expertise of medical doctors can play an important role in persuading audience behavioural intentions. Casting a non-celebrity medical doctor as a spokesperson may also have additional benefits. Research indicates that non-celebrity spokespersons, such as created characters, have the capacity to be more effective in producing memorability amongst audiences.[51] Furthermore, marketing doctors are given more freedom and control over limiting any associated risks, reducing the effect of multiple advertisement oversaturation,[52] and in reducing the chance of 'vampire effect' occurring; where the celebrity him- or herself can overshadow the advertisement message, leaving consumers remembering the spokesperson but not the actual endorsed product/message.[53] Given the potential risks and costs associated with use of celebrity spokespersons, as well as taking into account audience preferences matching the principles of many cancer charities that promote patient-centred care and consumer involvement in service planning, the results of this study suggest the use of medical doctor spokespersons for cancer prevention social marketing messages. Moreover, there is no additional benefit of using a celebrity doctor as health spokesperson.

## NOTES

1. R. Ohanian, 'The Impact of Celebrity Spokespersons' Perceived Image on Consumers' Intention to Purchase,' *Journal of Advertising Research* (1991): 460–54.
2. D.H. Silvera and B. Austad, 'Factors Predicting The Effectiveness Of Celebrity Endorsement Advertisements,' *European Journal of Marketing* 38, no. 11/12 (2004): 1509–26; L.R. Kahle and P.M. Homer, 'Physical Attractiveness of the Celebrity Endorser: A Social Adaptation Perspective,' *Journal of Consumer Research* 11, no. 4 (1985): 954–61; G.L. Patzer, 'Source Credibility as a Function of Communicator Physical Attractiveness,' *Journal of Business Research* 11, no. 2 (1983): 229–41; S.M. Petroshius and K.E. Crocker, 'An Empirical Analysis of Spokesperson Characteristics on Advertisement and Product Evaluations,' *Journal of the Academy of Marketing Science* 17, no. 3 (1989) 217–25; B.Y. Hakimi, A. Abedniya and M.N. Zaeim, 'Investigate the Impact of Celebrity Endorsement on Brand Image,' *European Journal of Scientific Research* 58, no. 1 (2011): 116–32; K. Chan, N. Yu Leung and E. K. Luk, 'Impact Of Celebrity Endorsement In Advertising On Brand Image Among Chinese Adolescents,' *Young Consumers* 14, no. 2 (2013): 167–79.
3. B. Casais and J.F. Proenca, 'Famous People Participation in Social Marketing Programs: A Research Focusing on Public Health,' *AMA Summer Educators Conference Proceeding: Enhancing Knowledge Development in Marketing* (2010): 516; N.W. Shead et al., 'Youth Gambling Prevention: Can Public Service Announcements Featuring Celebrity Spokespersons be Effective?' *International Journal of Mental Health & Addiction* 9, no. 2 (2011): 165–79; E. Samman, E. McAuliffe and M. MacLachlan, 'The Role Of Celebrity In Endorsing Poverty

Reduction Through International Aid,' *International Journal of Nonprofit and Voluntary Sector Marketing* 14, no. 2 (2009): 137–48; W. Wymer and T. Drollinger, 'Charity Appeals Using Celebrity Endorsers: Celebrity Attributes Most Predictive of Audience Donation Intentions,' *International Journal of Voluntary and Nonprofit Organizations* 26 (2015): 2694–717.

4. J. Ilicic and S. Baxter, 'Fit In Celebrity-Charity Alliances: When Perceived Celanthropy Benefits Nonprofit Organisations,' *International Journal of Nonprofit and Voluntary Sector Marketing* 19, no. 3 (2014): 200–8; R.T. Wheeler, 'Nonprofit Advertising: Impact of Celebrity Connection, Involvement and Gender on Source Credibility and Intention to Volunteer Time or Donate Money,' *Journal of Nonprofit & Public Sector Marketing* 21, no. 1 (2009): 80–107; M.d. M.G. de los Salmones, R. Dominguez and A. Herrero, 'Communication Using Celebrities in the Non-profit Sector: Determinants of its Effectiveness,' *International Journal of Advertising* 32, no. 1 (2013): 101–19; K. Panis and H. Van den Bulck, 'In The Footsteps Of Bob And Angelina: Celebrities' Diverse Societal Engagement And Its Ability To Attract Media Coverage,' *Communications: The European Journal of Communication Research* 39, no. 1 (2014): 23–42.

5. M.R. Stafford, T.F. Stafford and E. Day, 'A Contingency Approach: The Effects of Spokesperson Type and Service Type on Service Advertising Perceptions,' *Journal of Advertising* 31, no. 2 (2002): 17–35.

6. R. Ohanian, 'Construction and Validation of a Scale to Measure Celebrity Endorsers' Perceived Expertise, Trustworthiness, and Attractiveness,' *Journal of Advertising* 19, no. 3 (1990): 39–52; H.H. Friedman, M.J. Santeramo and A. Traina, 'Correlates Of Trustworthiness For Celebrities,' *Journal of the Academy of Marketing Science* 6, no. 4 (1978): 291–9; B. Sternthal, L.W. Phillips and R. Dholakia, 'The Persuasive Effect Of Source Credibility: A Situational Analysis,' *Public Opinion Quarterly* 42, no. 3 (1978): 285–314; N. Bhatt, R.M. Jayswal and J.D. Patel, 'Impact of Celebrity Endorser's Source Credibility on Attitude Towards Advertisements and Brands,' *South Asian Journal of Management* 20, no. 4 (2013): 74–95; E. McGinnies and C.D. Ward, 'Better Liked than Right: Trustworthiness and Expertise as Factors in Credibility,' *Personality and Social Psychology Bulletin* 6, no. 3 (1980): 467–72.

7. Ohanian, 'Construction and Validation,' 39–52; J.C. Siemens et al., 'Product Expertise Versus Professional Expertise: Congruency Between An Endorser's Chosen Profession And The Endorsed Product,' *Journal of Targeting, Measurement and Analysis for Marketing* 16, no. 3 (2008): 159–68.

8. Wheeler, 'Nonprofit Advertising,' 80–107; De los Salmones et al., 'Communication Using Celebrities,' 101–19; Stafford et al., 'A Contingency Approach,' 17–35; B.A. Lafferty and R.E. Goldsmith, 'Corporate Credibility's Role in Consumers' Attitudes and Purchase Intentions When a High versus a Low Credibility Endorser Is Used in the Ad,' *Journal of Business Research* 44 (1999): 109–16; H.H. Friedman, S. Termini and R. Washington, 'The Effectiveness of Advertisements Utilizing Four Types of Endorsers,' *Journal of Advertising* 5, no. 3 (1976): 22–4.

9. S. Michie et al., 'The Behavior Change Technique Taxonomy (v1) of 93 Hierarchially Clustered Techniques: Building an International Consensus for the Reporting of Behavior Change Interventions,' *Annuals of Behavioral Medicine* 46, no. 1 (2013): 81–95.

10. P. Koeppl and E. Robertson, 'The Healthy Choice: How Behavioral Factors Create Influential Health Campaign' (2015), available at: http://dupress.com/articles/behavior-change-communications-in-health-care/#end-notes; A.R. Andreasen, 'Social Marketing: Its Definition And Domain,' *Journal Of Public Policy & Marketing* 13, no. 1 (1994): 108–14; R. Gordon et al., 'The Effectiveness Of Social Marketing Interventions For Health Improvement: What's The Evidence?' *Public Health* 120, no. 12 (2006): 1133–9; M.A. Wakefield, B. Loken and R.C. Hornik, 'Use Of Mass Media Campaigns To Change Health Behaviour,' *The Lancet* 376, no. 9748 (2010): 1261–71; G.J.S. Wilde, 'Effects Of Mass Media Communications On Health And Safety Habits: An Overview Of Issues And Evidence,' *Addiction* 88, no. 7 (1993): 983–96.

11. C. Cox, '"Good For You TV": Using Storyboarding For Health-Related Television Public Service Announcements To Analyze Messages And Influence Positive Health Choices,' *The Journal of School Health* 78, no. 3 (2008): 179–83; W.R. Randolph and K. Viswanath, 'Lessons Learned From Public Health Mass Media Campaigns: Marketing Health In A Crowded Media World,' *Annual Review of Public Health* 25 (2004): 419–37.

12. M. Georgiadis, 'Motivating Behavior Change: A Content Analysis of Public Service Announcements From the Let's Move! Campaign,' *The Elon Journal of Undergraduate Research in Communications* 4, no. 1 (2013): 60–70; S.L. Brown and D. Whiting, 'The Ethics Of Distress: Toward A Framework For Determining The Ethical Acceptability Of Distressing Health Promotion Advertising,' *International Journal of Psychology* 49, no. 2 (2014): 89–97; M.R. Nelson et al., 'Get Real: How Current Behavior Influences Perceptions of Realism and Behavioral Intent for Public Service Announcements,' *Health Communication* 30, no. 7 (2014): 669–79.

13. National Health Service (NHS), 'Be Clear on Cancer' (2016), available at: http://www.nhs.uk/be-clear-on-cancer#7GZG3vGZrOzgCLpo.97; C. Bates, 'Persistent Cough "Could Be Warning Sign Of Lung Cancer": Stars Who Lost Relatives To Disease Launch Awareness Campaign' (2012), available at: http://www.dailymail.co.uk/health/article-2140644/Lung-cancer-symptoms-Persistent-cough-warning-sign.html#ixzz4EoAjxbgx; T. Knowles, '"Cough Campaign" Identifies 700 More Lung Cancer Patients' (2013), available at: https://www.thetimes.co.uk/article/cough-campaign-identifies-700-more-lung-cancer-patients-czsvbqnbbw5; Gov.UK. '"Don't Ignore A Persistent Cough," Warns Lung Cancer Campaign' (2013), available at: https://www.gov.uk/government/news/dont-ignore-a-persistent-cough-warns-lung-cancer-campaign; Cancer Research UK. 'About Be Clear on Cancer' (2014), available at: http://www.cancerresearchuk.org/health-professional/early-diagnosis-activities/be-clear-on-cancer/about-be-clear-on-cancer#BCOC_about0.

14. J.D. Newton, J. Wong and F.J. Newton, 'The Social Status of Health Message Endorsers Influences the Health Intentions of the Powerless,' *Journal of Advertising* 44, no. 2 (2015): 151–60; K. Braunsberger and J. M. Munch, 'Source Expertise Versus Experience Effects In Hospital Advertising,' *Journal of Services Marketing* 12, no. 1 (1998): 23–38; Y. Hu and S. Sundar, 'Effects of Online Health Sources on Credibility and Behavioral Intentions,' *Communications Research* 37, no. 1 (2010): 1–28; A.J. Bush, W.C. Moncrief and V.A. Ziethaml, 'Source Effects in Professional Services Advertising,' *Current Issues & Research in Advertising* 10, no. 1 (1987): 153.

15. Friedman et al., 'The Effectiveness of Advertisements,' 22–4.

16. D. Biswas, A. Biswas and N. Das, 'The Differential Effects of Celebrity and Expert Endorsements on Consumer Risk Perceptions. The Role of Consumer Knowledge, Perceived Congruency, and Product Technology Orientation,' *Journal of Advertising* 35, no. 2 (2006): 17–31.

17. Roy Morgan Research, 'Roy Morgan Image Of Professions Survey 2015–Nurses Still Easily Most Highly Regarded–Followed By Doctors, Pharmacists & School Teachers' (2015), available at: http://www.roymorgan.com/findings/6188-roy-morgan-image-of-professions-2015-201504280343.

18. IPSOS-MORI, 'Politicians Are Still Trusted Less Than Estate Agents, Journalists And Bankers' (2016), available at: https://www.ipsos-mori.com/researchpublications/researcharchive/3685/Politicians-are-still-trusted-less-than-estate-agents-journalists-and-bankers.aspx.

19. Braunsberger and Munch, 'Source Expertise,' 23–38; H.H. Friedman and L. Friedman, 'Endorser Effectiveness by Product Type,' *Journal of Advertising Research* 19, no. 5 (1979): 63–71; C.I. Hovland, I.L. Janis

and H.H. Kelley, *Communication And Persuasion: Psychological Studies Of Opinion Change* (Santa Barbara, CA: Greenwood Press, 1953); B.Z. Erdogan, 'Celebrity Endorsement: A Literature Review,' *Journal of Marketing Management* 15, no. 3 (1999): 291–314.

20. Biswas et al., 'The Differential Effects,' 17–31; R. Crisci and H. Kassinove, 'Effect of Perceived Expertise, Strength of Advice, and Environmental Setting on Parental Compliance,' *Journal of Social Psychology* 89, no. 2 (1973): 245–50.

21. W.D. Crano, 'Effects of Sex, Response Order, and Expertise in Conformity: A Dispositional Approach,' *Sociometry* 33, no. 3 (1970): 239–52.

22. V. Klucharev, A. Smidts and G. Fernández, 'Brain Mechanisms Of Persuasion: How "Expert Power" Modulates Memory And Attitudes,' *Social Cognitive and Affective Neuroscience* 3, no. 4 (2008): 353–66; R.D. Stainback and R.W. Rogers, 'Identifying Effective Components of Alcohol Abuse Prevention Programs: Effects of Fear Appeals, Message Style, and Source Expertise,' *International Journal of the Addictions* 18, no. 3 (1983): 393–405; M.R. Durantini et al., 'Conceptualizing the Influence of Social Agents of Behavior Change: A Meta-Analysis of the Effectiveness of HIV-Prevention Interventionists for Different Groups,' *Psychological Bulletin* 132, no. 2 (2006): 212–48.

23. Hu and Sundar, 'Effects of Online Health Sources,' 1–28.

24. Braunsberger and Munch, 'Source Expertise,' 23–38.

25. Friedman et al., 'The Effectiveness of Advertisements,' 22–4; Friedman and Friedman, 'Endorser Effectiveness,' 63–71; R.J. Larson et al., 'Celebrity Endorsements of Cancer Screening,' *Journal of the National Cancer Institute* 97, no. 9 (2005): 693–5.

26. Friedman and Friedman, 'Endorser Effectiveness,' 63–71.

27. Stafford et al., 'A Contingency Effect,' 17–35; Erdogan, 'Celebrity Endorsement,' 291; S.J. Hoffman and C. Tan, 'Following Celebrities' Medical Advice: Meta-Narrative Analysis,' *British Medical Journal* 347 (2013): 7151; A. Spry, R. Pappu and T.B. Cornwell, 'Celebrity Endorsement, Brand Credibility And Brand Equity,' *European Journal of Marketing* 45, no. 6 (2011): 882–909; J.W. Ayers et al., 'Do Celebrity Cancer Diagnoses Promote Primary Cancer Prevention?' *Preventive Medicine* 58 (2014): 81–4.

28. Ohanian, 'Construction and Validation,' 39–52; Friedman and Friedman, 'Endorser Effectiveness,' 63–71; Hovland et al., *Communication and Persuasion*; J.M. Kamen, A.C. Azhari and J.R. Kragh, 'What a Spokesman Does for a Sponsor,' *Journal of Advertising Research* 15, no. 2 (1975): 17–24; C. Atkin and M. Block, 'Effectiveness of Celebrity Endorsers,' *Journal of Advertising Research* 23, no. 1 (1983): 57–61; G. McCracken,

'Who is the Celebrity Endorser? Cultural Foundations of the Endorsement Process,' *Journal of Consumer Research* 16, no. 3 (1989): 310–21.

29. Biswas et al., 'The Differential Effects,' 17–31; J.B. Freiden, 'Advertising Spokesperson Effects: An Examination of Endorser Type and Gender on Two Audiences,' *Journal of Advertising Research* 24, no. 5 (1984): 33; B.D. Till and M. Busler, 'Matching Products With Endorsers: Attractiveness Versus Expertise,' *Journal of Consumer Marketing* 15, no. 6 (1998): 576–86.

30. R.E. Petty, J.T. Cacioppo and D. Schumann, 'Central And Peripheral Routes To Advertising Effectiveness: The Moderating Role Of Involvement,' *Journal of Consumer Research* 10, no. 2 (1983): 135–46.

31. R.A. Swerdlow and M.R. Swerdlow, 'Celebrity Endorsers: Spokesperson Selection Criteria And Case Examples Of FREDD,' *Academy Of Marketing Studies Journal* 7, no. 2 (2003): 13–26.

32. Ibid; Siemans et al., 'Product Expertise,' 159–68; Erdogan, 'Celebrity Endoresement,' 291–314; McCracken, 'Who Is the Celebrity Endorser?' 310–21; M.A. Kamins and K. Gupta, 'Congruence between Spokesperson and Product Type: A Matchup Hypothesis Perspective.' *Psychology & Marketing* 11, no. 6 (1994): 569–86.

33. Chan et al., 'Impact of Celebrity Endorsement,' 167–79.

34. Shead et al., 'Youth Gambling Prevention,' 165–79; S. Chapman and J.-A. Leask, 'Paid Celebrity Endorsement in Health Promotion: A Case Study,' *Health Promotion International* 16 (2001): 333–8; W.-C. Tsai et al. 'Effects Of A Tobacco Prevention Education Program On Adolescents' Knowledge Of And Attitude Toward Smoking,' *Mid-Taiwan Journal of Medicine* 10, no. 4 (2005): 171–80; T. Seghers and S. Foland, 'Anti-Tobacco Media Campaign For Young People,' *Tobacco Control* 7 (s1) (1998): S29–S30; W. DeJong and C.K. Atkin, 'A Review of National Television PSA Campaigns for Preventing Alcohol-Impaired Driving, 1987–1992,' *Journal of Public Health Policy* 16, no. 1 (1995): 59–81.

35. N. Bootsman, D.F. Blackburn and J. Taylor, 'The Oz Craze: The Effect Of Pop Culture Media On Health Care,' *Canadian Pharmacists Journal* 147, no. 2 (2014): 80–2; J. F. Hagenbruch, 'Dr. Oz Sells Out The Hippocratic Oath,' *CDS Review* 106, no. 7 (2013): 5; C. Korownyk et al., 'Televised Medical Talk Shows—What They Recommend And The Evidence To Support Their Recommendations: A Prospective Observational Study,' *British Medical Journal* 349, no. 9 (2014): doi:10.1136/bmj.g7346.

36. Department of Health, 'The Expert Patient: A New Approach To Chronic Disease Management For The 21st Century,' (London: Department of Health, 2001); R.E. Say and R. Thomson, 'The

Importance Of Patient Preferences In Treatment Decisions—Challenges For Doctors,' *British Medical Journal* 327 (2003): 542–5; A.C. Mühlbacher and C. Juhnke, 'Patient Preferences Versus Physicians' Judgement: Does It Make A Difference In Healthcare Decision Making?' *Applied Health Economics and Health Policy* 11, no. 3 (2013): 163–80.

37. A. Coulter, S. Parsons and J. Askham, 'Health Systems And Policy Analysis: Where Are The Patients On Decision-Making About Their Own Care?' in *WHO European Ministerial Conference on Health Systems: "Health Systems, Health and Wealth–."* (Tallinn, Estonia: World Health Organization, 2008).

38. Research Now. *Research Now* (2016), available at: https://www.research-now.com/.

39. F. Faul et al., 'G*Power 3: A Flexible Statistical Power Analysis Program For The Social, Behavioral, And Biomedical Sciences,' *Behavior Research Methods* 39, no. 2 (2007): 175–91.

40. Ohanian, 'Construction and Validation,' 39–52.

41. Wheeler, 'Nonprofit Advertising,' 80–107.

42. H.A. Taute, S. McQuitty and E.P. Sautter, 'Emotional Information Management and Responses to Emotional Appeals,' *Journal of Advertising* 40, no. 3 (2011): 31–43.

43. Wheeler, Nonprofit Advertising,' 80–107; Illicic and Baxter, 'Fit in Celebrity-Charity Alliances,' 200–8.

44. B. Rollins and N. Bhutada, 'Impact Of Celebrity Endorsements In Disease-Specific Direct-To-Consumer (DTC) Advertisements: An Elaboration Likelihood Model Approach,' *International Journal of Pharmaceutical and Healthcare Marketing* 8, no. 2 (2014): 164–77.

45. A.P.J. Matheny, R.S. Wilson and A.B. Dolan, 'Relations Between Twins' Similarity of Appearance and Behavioral Similarity: Testing an Assumption,' *Behavior Genetics* 6, no. 3 (1976): 343–51.

46. Cancer Council SA, *Are you SunSmart?* in *Flyer*, Cancer Council SA (2015), Cancer Council South Australia, Online; Cancer Council Victoria. 'Welcome to SunSmart' (2017), available at: http://www.sunsmart.com.au/.

47. Ohanian, 'Construction and Validation,' 39–52; Friedman and Friedman, 'Endorser Effectiveness,' 63–71; Hovland et al., *Communication and Persuasion*.

48. De Los Salmones et al., 'Communication Using Celebrities,' 101–19; McGinnies and Ward, 'Better Liked than Right,' 467–72; M. Eisend and T. Langner, 'Immediate And Delayed Advertising Effects Of Celebrity Endorsers' Attractiveness And Expertise,' *International Journal of Advertising* 29, no. 4 (2010): 527–46.

49. Braunsberger and Munch, 'Source Expertise,' 23–38; Hu and Sundar, 'Effects of Online Health Sources,' 1–28.
50. Ohanian, 'Construction and Validation,' 39–52; Friedman et al., 'Correlates of Trustworthiness,' 291–9; Friedman and Friedman, 'Endorser Effectiveness,' 63–71; Hovland et al., *Communication and Persuasion*; Erdogan, 'Celebrity Endorsement,' 291–314.
51. G. Tom et al., 'The Use Of Created Versus Celebrity Spokespersons In Advertisements,' *Journal of Consumer Marketing* 9, no. 4 (1992): 45–51.
52. Ibid.
53. Bhatt et al., 'Impact of Celebrity,' 74–95; Erdogan, 'Celebrity Endorsement,' 291–314.

**Acknowledgements** This research has received a statistical support grant from the Hunter Cancer Research Alliance (HCRA). HCRA receives funding from the Cancer Institute NSW to operate as a Translational Cancer Research Centre, the University of Newcastle and the Hunter Medical Research Institute.

Acknowledgement to Cancer Council South Australia for the original development of the resource used in the study, and for the guidance and cooperation of Cancer Council NSW in supporting the study. Use of the SunSmart Program logo has been reproduced with the permission of the SunSmart Program at Cancer Council Victoria.

# REFERENCES

Andreasen, A.R. 'Social Marketing: Its Definition And Domain.' *Journal Of Public Policy & Marketing* 13, no. 1 (1994): 108–14.

Atkin, C. and M. Block. 'Effectiveness of Celebrity Endorsers.' *Journal of Advertising Research* 23, no. 1 (1983): 57–61.

Ayers, J.W. et al. 'Do Celebrity Cancer Diagnoses Promote Primary Cancer Prevention?' *Preventive Medicine* 58 (2014): 81–4.

Bates, C. 'Persistent Cough "Could Be Warning Sign Of Lung Cancer": Stars Who Lost Relatives To Disease Launch Awareness Campaign.' (2012), available at: http://www.dailymail.co.uk/health/article-2140644/Lung-cancer-symptoms-Persistent-cough-warning-sign.html#ixzz4EoAjxbgx.

Bhatt, N., R.M. Jayswal and J.D. Patel. 'Impact of Celebrity Endorser's Source Credibility on Attitude Towards Advertisements and Brands.' *South Asian Journal of Management* 20, no. 4 (2013): 74–95.

Biswas, D., A. Biswas and N. Das. 'The Differential Effects of Celebrity and Expert Endorsements on Consumer Risk Perceptions. The Role of Consumer Knowledge, Perceived Congruency, and Product Technology Orientation.' *Journal of Advertising* 35, no. 2 (2006): 17–31.

Bootsman, N., D.F. Blackburn and J. Taylor. 'The Oz Craze: The Effect Of Pop Culture Media On Health Care.' *Canadian Pharmacists Journal* 147, no. 2 (2014): 80–2.

Braunsberger, K. and J.M. Munch. 'Source Expertise Versus Experience Effects In Hospital Advertising.' *Journal of Services Marketing* 12, no. 1 (1998): 23–38.

Brown, S.L. and D. Whiting. 'The Ethics Of Distress: Toward A Framework For Determining The Ethical Acceptability Of Distressing Health Promotion Advertising.' *International Journal of Psychology* 49, no. 2 (2014): 89–97.

Bush, A.J., W.C. Moncrief and V.A. Ziethaml. 'Source Effects in Professional Services Advertising.' *Current Issues & Research in Advertising* 10, no. 1 (1987): 153.

Cancer Council SA. *Are you SunSmart?* in *Flyer*, Cancer Council SA (2015), Cancer Council South Australia, Online; Cancer Council Victoria. 'Welcome to SunSmart.' (2017), available at: http://www.sunsmart.com.au/.

Cancer Research UK. 'About Be Clear on Cancer.' (2014), available at: http://www.cancerresearchuk.org/health-professional/early-diagnosis-activities/be-clear-on-cancer/about-be-clear-on-cancer#BCOC_about0.

Casais, B. and J.F. Proenca. 'Famous People Participation in Social Marketing Programs: A Research Focusing on Public Health.' *AMA Summer Educators Conference Proceeding: Enhancing Knowledge Development in Marketing* (2010): 516.

Chan, K., N. Yu Leung and E.K. Luk. 'Impact Of Celebrity Endorsement In Advertising On Brand Image Among Chinese Adolescents.' *Young Consumers* 14, no. 2 (2013): 167–79.

Chapman, S. and J.-A. Leask. 'Paid Celebrity Endorsement in Health Promotion: A Case Study.' *Health Promotion International* 16 (2001): 333–8.

Coulter, A., S. Parsons and J. Askham. 'Health Systems And Policy Analysis: Where Are The Patients On Decision-Making About Their Own Care?' in *WHO European Ministerial Conference on Health Systems: "Health Systems, Health and Wealth."* (Tallinn, Estonia: World Health Organization, 2008).

Cox, C. '"Good For You TV": Using Storyboarding For Health-Related Television Public Service Announcements To Analyze Messages And Influence Positive Health Choices.' *The Journal of School Health* 78, no. 3 (2008): 179–83.

Crano, W.D. 'Effects of Sex, Response Order, and Expertise in Conformity: A Dispositional Approach.' *Sociometry* 33, no. 3 (1970): 239–52.

Crisci, R. and H. Kassinove. 'Effect of Perceived Expertise, Strength of Advice, and Environmental Setting on Parental Compliance.' *Journal of Social Psychology* 89, no. 2 (1973): 245–50.

DeJong, W. and C.K. Atkin. 'A Review of National Television PSA Campaigns for Preventing Alcohol-Impaired Driving, 1987–1992.' *Journal of Public Health Policy* 16, no. 1 (1995): 59–81.

de los Salmones, M.d. M.G., R. Dominguez and A. Herrero. 'Communication Using Celebrities in the Non-profit Sector: Determinants of its Effectiveness.' *International Journal of Advertising* 32, no. 1 (2013): 101–19.

Department of Health. 'The Expert Patient: A New Approach To Chronic Disease Management For The 21st Century.' (London: Department of Health, 2001).

Durantini, M.R. et al. 'Conceptualizing the Influence of Social Agents of Behavior Change: A Meta-Analysis of the Effectiveness of HIV-Prevention Interventionists for Different Groups.' *Psychological Bulletin* 132, no. 2 (2006): 212–48.

Eisend, M. and T. Langner. 'Immediate And Delayed Advertising Effects Of Celebrity Endorsers' Attractiveness And Expertise.' *International Journal of Advertising* 29, no. 4 (2010): 527–46.

Erdogan, B.Z. 'Celebrity Endorsement: A Literature Review.' *Journal of Marketing Management* 15, no. 3 (1999): 291–314.

Faul, F. et al. 'G*Power 3: A Flexible Statistical Power Analysis Program For The Social, Behavioral, And Biomedical Sciences.' *Behavior Research Methods* 39, no. 2 (2007): 175–91.

Freiden, J.B. 'Advertising Spokesperson Effects: An Examination of Endorser Type and Gender on Two Audiences.' *Journal of Advertising Research* 24, no. 5 (1984): 33.

Friedman, H.H. and L. Friedman. 'Endorser Effectiveness by Product Type.' *Journal of Advertising Research* 19, no. 5 (1979): 63–71.

Friedman, H.H., M.J. Santeramo and A. Traina. 'Correlates Of Trustworthiness For Celebrities.' *Journal of the Academy of Marketing Science* 6, no. 4 (1978): 291–9.

Friedman, H.H., S. Termini and R. Washington. 'The Effectiveness of Advertisements Utilizing Four Types of Endorsers.' *Journal of Advertising* 5, no. 3 (1976): 22–4.

Georgiadis. M. 'Motivating Behavior Change: A Content Analysis of Public Service Announcements From the Let's Move! Campaign.' *The Elon Journal of Undergraduate Research in Communications* 4, no. 1 (2013): 60–70.

Gordon, R. et al. 'The Effectiveness Of Social Marketing Interventions For Health Improvement: What's The Evidence?' *Public Health* 120, no. 12 (2006): 1133–9.

Gov.UK. '"Don't Ignore A Persistent Cough," Warns Lung Cancer Campaign.' (2013), available at: https://www.gov.uk/government/news/dont-ignore-a-persistent-cough-warns-lung-cancer-campaign.

Hagenbruch, J.F. 'Dr. Oz Sells Out The Hippocratic Oath.' *CDS Review* 106, no. 7 (2013): 5.

Hakimi, B.Y., A. Abedniya and M.N. Zaeim. 'Investigate the Impact of Celebrity Endorsement on Brand Image.' *European Journal of Scientific Research* 58, no. 1 (2011): 116–32.

Hoffman, S.J. and C. Tan. 'Following Celebrities' Medical Advice: Meta-Narrative Analysis.' *British Medical Journal* 347 (2013): 7151.

Hovland, C.I., I.L. Janis and H.H. Kelley, *Communication And Persuasion: Psychological Studies Of Opinion Change.* Santa Barbara, CA: Greenwood Press, 1953.

Hu, Y. and S. Sundar. 'Effects of Online Health Sources on Credibility and Behavioral Intentions.' *Communications Research* 37, no. 1 (2010): 1–28.

Ilicic, J. and S. Baxter. 'Fit In Celebrity-Charity Alliances: When Perceived Celanthropy Benefits Nonprofit Organisations.' *International Journal of Nonprofit and Voluntary Sector Marketing* 19, no. 3 (2014): 200–8.

IPSOS-MORI, 'Politicians Are Still Trusted Less Than Estate Agents, Journalists And Bankers.' (2016), available at: https://www.ipsos-mori.com/research-publications/researcharchive/3685/Politicians-are-still-trusted-less-than-estate-agents-journalists-and-bankers.aspx.

Kahle, L.R. and P.M. Homer. 'Physical Attractiveness of the Celebrity Endorser: A Social Adaptation Perspective.' *Journal of Consumer Research* 11, no. 4 (1985): 954–61.

Kamen, J.M., A.C. Azhari and J.R. Kragh. 'What a Spokesman Does for a Sponsor.' *Journal of Advertising Research* 15, no. 2 (1975): 17–24.

Kamins, M.A. and K. Gupta. 'Congruence between Spokesperson and Product Type: A Matchup Hypothesis Perspective.' *Psychology & Marketing* 11, no. 6 (1994): 569–86.

Klucharev, V., A. Smidts and G. Fernández, 'Brain Mechanisms Of Persuasion: How "Expert Power" Modulates Memory And Attitudes.' *Social Cognitive and Affective Neuroscience* 3, no. 4 (2008): 353–66.

Knowles, T. '"Cough Campaign" Identifies 700 More Lung Cancer Patients.' (2013), available at: https://www.thetimes.co.uk/article/cough-campaign-identifies-700-more-lung-cancer-patients-czsvbqnbbw5.

Koeppl, P. and E. Robertson. 'The Healthy Choice: How Behavioral Factors Create Influential Health Campaign.' (2015), available at: http://dupress.com/articles/behavior-change-communications-in-health-care/#end-notes.

Korownyk, C. et al. 'Televised Medical Talk Shows—What They Recommend And The Evidence To Support Their Recommendations: A Prospective Observational Study.' *British Medical Journal* 349, no. 9 (2014): doi: 10.1136/bmj.g7346.

Lafferty, B.A. and R.E. Goldsmith. 'Corporate Credibility's Role in Consumers' Attitudes and Purchase Intentions When a High versus a Low Credibility Endorser Is Used in the Ad.' *Journal of Business Research* 44 (1999): 109–16.

Larson, R.J. et al. 'Celebrity Endorsements of Cancer Screening.' *Journal of the National Cancer Institute* 97, no. 9 (2005): 693–5.

Matheny, A.P.J., R.S. Wilson and A.B. Dolan. 'Relations Between Twins' Similarity of Appearance and Behavioral Similarity: Testing an Assumption.' *Behavior Genetics* 6, no. 3 (1976): 343–51.

McCracken, G. 'Who is the Celebrity Endorser? Cultural Foundations of the Endorsement Process.' *Journal of Consumer Research* 16, no. 3 (1989): 310–21.

McGinnies E. and C.D. Ward. 'Better Liked than Right: Trustworthiness and Expertise as Factors in Credibility.' *Personality and Social Psychology Bulletin* 6, no. 3 (1980): 467–72.

Michie, S. et al. 'The Behavior Change Technique Taxonomy (v1) of 93 Hierarchially Clustered Techniques: Building an International Consensus for the Reporting of Behavior Change Interventions.' *Annuals of Behavioral Medicine* 46, no. 1 (2013): 81–95.

Mühlbacher, A.C. and C. Juhnke. 'Patient Preferences Versus Physicians' Judgement: Does It Make A Difference In Healthcare Decision Making?' *Applied Health Economics and Health Policy* 11, no. 3 (2013): 163–80.

National Health Service (NHS). 'Be Clear on Cancer.' (2016), available at: http://www.nhs.uk/be-clear-on-cancer#7GZG3vGZrOzgCLpo.97.

Nelson, M.R. et al. 'Get Real: How Current Behavior Influences Perceptions of Realism and Behavioral Intent for Public Service Announcements.' *Health Communication* 30, no. 7 (2014): 669–79.

Newton, J.D., J. Wong and F.J. Newton. 'The Social Status of Health Message Endorsers Influences the Health Intentions of the Powerless.' *Journal of Advertising* 44, no. 2 (2015): 151–60.

Ohanian, R. 'The Impact of Celebrity Spokespersons' Perceived Image on Consumers' Intention to Purchase.' *Journal of Advertising Research* (1991): 460–54.

———. 'Construction and Validation of a Scale to Measure Celebrity Endorsers' Perceived Expertise, Trustworthiness, and Attractiveness,' *Journal of Advertising* 19, no. 3 (1990): 39–52.

Panis, K. and H. Van den Bulck. 'In The Footsteps Of Bob And Angelina: Celebrities' Diverse Societal Engagement And Its Ability To Attract Media Coverage.' *Communications: The European Journal of Communication Research* 39, no. 1 (2014): 23–42.

Patzer, G.L. 'Source Credibility as a Function of Communicator Physical Attractiveness.' *Journal of Business Research* 11, no. 2 (1983): 229–41.

Petroshius, S.M. and K.E. Crocker. 'An Empirical Analysis of Spokesperson Characteristics on Advertisement and Product Evaluations.' *Journal of the Academy of Marketing Science* 17, no. 3 (1989): 217–25.

Petty, R.E., J.T. Cacioppo and D. Schumann. 'Central And Peripheral Routes To Advertising Effectiveness: The Moderating Role Of Involvement.' *Journal of Consumer Research* 10, no. 2 (1983): 135–46.

Randolph, W.R. and K. Viswanath, 'Lessons Learned From Public Health Mass Media Campaigns: Marketing Health In A Crowded Media World.' *Annual Review of Public Health* 25 (2004): 419–37.

Research Now. *Research Now.* (2016), available at: https://www.researchnow.com/.

Rollins, B. and N. Bhutada. 'Impact Of Celebrity Endorsements In Disease-Specific Direct-To-Consumer (DTC) Advertisements: An Elaboration Likelihood Model Approach.' *International Journal of Pharmaceutical and Healthcare Marketing* 8, no. 2 (2014): 164–77.

Roy Morgan Research. 'Roy Morgan Image Of Professions Survey 2015 – Nurses Still Easily Most Highly Regarded – Followed By Doctors, Pharmacists & School Teachers.' (2015), available at: http://www.roymorgan.com/findings/6188-roy-morgan-image-of-profesions-2015-201504280343.

Samman, E. E. McAuliffe and M. MacLachlan. 'The Role Of Celebrity In Endorsing Poverty Reduction Through International Aid.' *International Journal of Nonprofit and Voluntary Sector Marketing* 14, no. 2 (2009): 137–48.

Say, R.E. and R. Thomson. 'The Importance Of Patient Preferences In Treatment Decisions—Challenges For Doctors.' *British Medical Journal* 327 (2003): 542–5.

Seghers, T. and S. Foland. 'Anti-Tobacco Media Campaign For Young People.' *Tobacco Control* 7 (s1) (1998): S29–S30.

Shead, N.W. et al. 'Youth Gambling Prevention: Can Public Service Announcements Featuring Celebrity Spokespersons be Effective?' *International Journal of Mental Health & Addiction* 9, no. 2 (2011): 165–79.

Siemens, J.C. et al. 'Product Expertise Versus Professional Expertise: Congruency Between An Endorser's Chosen Profession And The Endorsed Product.' *Journal of Targeting, Measurement and Analysis for Marketing* 16, no. 3 (2008): 159–68.

Silvera, D.H. and B. Austad. 'Factors Predicting The Effectiveness Of Celebrity Endorsement Advertisements.' *European Journal of Marketing* 38, no. 11/12 (2004): 1509–26.

Spry, A., R. Pappu and T.B. Cornwell. 'Celebrity Endorsement, Brand Credibility And Brand Equity.' *European Journal of Marketing* 45, no. 6 (2011): 882–909.

Stafford, M.R., T.F. Stafford and E. Day. 'A Contingency Approach: The Effects of Spokesperson Type and Service Type on Service Advertising Perceptions.' *Journal of Advertising* 31, no. 2 (2002): 17–35.

Stainback, R.D. and R.W. Rogers. 'Identifying Effective Components of Alcohol Abuse Prevention Programs: Effects of Fear Appeals, Message Style, and Source Expertise.' *International Journal of the Addictions* 18, no. 3 (1983): 393–405.

Sternthal, B., L.W. Phillips and R. Dholakia. 'The Persuasive Effect Of Source Credibility: A Situational Analysis.' *Public Opinion Quarterly* 42, no. 3 (1978): 285–314.

Swerdlow, R.A. and M.R. Swerdlow. 'Celebrity Endorsers: Spokesperson Selection Criteria And Case Examples Of FREDD.' *Academy Of Marketing Studies Journal* 7, no. 2 (2003): 13–26.

Taute, H.A., S. McQuitty and E.P. Sautter. 'Emotional Information Management and Responses to Emotional Appeals.' *Journal of Advertising* 40, no. 3 (2011): 31–43.

Till, B.D. and M. Busler. 'Matching Products With Endorsers: Attractiveness Versus Expertise.' *Journal of Consumer Marketing* 15, no. 6 (1998): 576–86.

Tom, G. et al. 'The Use Of Created Versus Celebrity Spokespersons In Advertisements.' *Journal of Consumer Marketing* 9, no. 4 (1992): 45–51.

Tsai, W.-C. et al. 'Effects Of A Tobacco Prevention Education Program On Adolescents' Knowledge Of And Attitude Toward Smoking.' *Mid-Taiwan Journal of Medicine* 10, no. 4 (2005): 171–80.

Wakefield, M.A., B. Loken and R.C. Hornik. 'Use Of Mass Media Campaigns To Change Health Behaviour.' *The Lancet* 376, no. 9748 (2010): 1261–71.

Wheeler, R.T. 'Nonprofit Advertising: Impact of Celebrity Connection, Involvement and Gender on Source Credibility and Intention to Volunteer Time or Donate Money.' *Journal of Nonprofit & Public Sector Marketing* 21, no. 1 (2009): 80–107.

Wilde, G.J.S. 'Effects Of Mass Media Communications On Health And Safety Habits: An Overview Of Issues And Evidence.' *Addiction* 88, no. 7 (1993): 983–96.

Wymer W. and T. Drollinger. 'Charity Appeals Using Celebrity Endorsers: Celebrity Attributes Most Predictive of Audience Donation Intentions.' *International Journal of Voluntary and Nonprofit Organizations* 26 (2015): 2694–717.

# An Empirical Study of Student Engagement with Professional and Ethical Issues in Medical Television Dramas

## Evie Kendal and Basia Diug

Why students opt to pursue medicine as a career has been the subject of much scholarly debate. Historically, theorists such as G.S. Becker (1962) and Bernard Lentz and David Laband (1989) have attributed many cases to 'human capital formation' within the family unit.[1] To summarise Lentz and Laband's argument, the children of doctors experience an intergenerational transfer of career-specific human capital that motivates them to voluntarily pursue a career in medicine and also better prepares them for pursuing this course of study. While it may still be true that there are a disproportionate number of doctors' children successfully applying to medical school in the 21st century, as in the 20th, the purpose of this project was to engage with other motivating factors that inspire students to enrol in medicine and allied health degrees. Specifically, we were interested in exploring the impact of popular culture

E. Kendal (✉) · B. Diug
Monash University, Melbourne, Australia
e-mail: evie.kendal@monash.edu

B. Diug
e-mail: basia.diug@monash.edu

© The Author(s) 2017
E. Kendal and B. Diug (eds.), *Teaching Medicine and Medical Ethics Using Popular Culture*, Palgrave Studies in Science and Popular Culture, DOI 10.1007/978-3-319-65451-5_6

on the perception of medical studies and careers, and whether this too may motivate and prepare future doctors and allied health professionals. If accepting that a parent can serve as a role model for a future doctor, it seems reasonable to hypothesise that a fictional character may function as a substitute role model for students who may not have doctors or health professionals in their families. Furthermore, we wanted to gauge our students' exposure to popular medical television and their perception of its pedagogical value in medical education.

It is known that medical and nursing students watch medical television dramas and comedies. Matthew J. Czarny et al.'s study from Johns Hopkins University in 2008 cites 84% of medical students and 81% of nursing students surveyed reported watching medical television dramas.[2] Roslyn Weaver and Ian Wilson repeated this study in Australia in 2011, finding 93.7% of medical students reported watching medical dramas.[3] Among the shows specifically mentioned in these studies were *Grey's Anatomy*, *House M.D.*, *Scrubs* and *ER*. The above data indicates that incorporating popular culture references into medical and health education is likely to increase student engagement, and represents a source of untapped potential for effective communication of medical information from lecturers to students and, further downstream, from doctors to patients. Medical teaching facilities engaging with this form of education have reported consistently positive results, from students and tutors.[4]

Weaver and Wilson claim that medically focused popular culture is particularly well poised to assist in the communication of ethical and professional issues affecting clinicians, but that it needs to be approached in such a way as to ensure students receive an 'authentic perception' of the career they are entering.[5] These results are supported by Anna Pavlov and Gregory Dahlquist's 2010 study of medical residents, who reported that the use of movie clips in clinical education was useful for stimulating interest and setting the scene for case discussions, but that clear learning objectives needed to be established for them.[6]

According to Gladys B. White, the popularity of medical television dramas for medicine and health science students is connected to their personal anxieties about their chosen profession, including how they will perform under pressure or achieve work–life balance. Although she claims the issues surrounding the delivery of healthcare in many of these shows are 'somewhat self-centred' from the perspective of the caregivers, these concerns are the same ones plaguing future doctors and health professionals.[7] As such, the opportunity to observe and learn from the experiences of a fictional healthcare provider may be particularly valuable for students as they develop their clinical and professional skills. Previous research also shows that popular media representations of careers not only impact recruitment and retention in these areas of study, but may also help students form their professional identities early in their studies.[8]

The aim of this study was to investigate how medical students and those enrolled in other health-related university degrees engaged with popular culture, and particularly medical television dramas. Points of interest included how accurate students thought these programmes were, whether they sourced professional role models from these fictional sources, how appropriately they thought television writers handled sensitive ethical issues in their stories, and whether they thought popular culture representations influenced their own opinions, those of their family or friends, or policymakers involved in healthcare decision-making.

## METHOD

A modified and updated version of the pre-validated questionnaire used in Weaver and Wilson's study from 2011 was used in this project, which was itself adapted from the one used in Matthew J. Czarny et al.'s study of 2008. This questionnaire asked students to record their level of exposure to popular medical television, their perception of the accuracy of these shows and whether or not they wanted to be like any of the characters depicted. Based on the future research recommendations of these authors, we extended the research cohort to include biomedical and health science students in addition to medical students, to provide another source of comparison. The study used a cross-sectional design with a partially open (i.e. free-form comments) and partially closed (i.e. yes/no) question survey, intended to provide both quantitative and qualitative data. The qualitative data was descriptive, while most of the quantitative data was collected through Likert scales (in which students selected strongly agree, agree, neutral, disagree or strongly disagree in response to a particular survey item or statement). The paper questionnaire was administered in tutorials for first year students in Monash University's Bachelor of Medicine/Bachelor of Surgery (MBBS), Bachelor of Biomedical Science (BMS) and Bachelor of Health Science (HSC) degree programmes. The study was run in the second semester of 2015 at both the Clayton and Caulfield campuses in Victoria, Australia.

Weaver and Wilson's study is thus a particularly valuable comparator as it also focused on students at an Australian university.

The MBBS is a five-year undergraduate medical degree, qualifying students to practise as doctors within the Australian healthcare sector. This degree accepts students directly after completing high school, contrasting the graduate medical programme that recruits students who have already completed a first degree. The MBBS programme consists of classroom learning and clinical placements. The BMS degree is a three-year undergraduate programme, which incorporates theory and laboratory classes on the topic of human biological systems. Graduates of the BMS degree can apply for graduate medicine programmes, research degrees or undertake further practical studies in health, for example, radiography. The HSC degree is also a three-year undergraduate programme, focused on public health and policy. It does not typically involve laboratory classes. There are no clinical placements in either the BMS or HSC degree, although some students complete research projects attached to hospitals.

Ethics approval for this study was granted by the Monash University Human Research Ethics Committee and all data was collected anonymously. Participation was voluntary and students completed the questionnaires on an opt-in basis.

## RESULTS

Of the 902 students invited to participate in the study, 664 students completed a questionnaire that was eligible for inclusion in the study. This equates to a response rate of 73.6%. Of these 664 students, 114 (17%) were from the Bachelor of Health Sciences (HSC), representing 88% of this cohort, 286 (43%) were from the Bachelor of Biomedical Sciences (BMS), representing 61% of this cohort, and 264 (40%) were enrolled in the Bachelor of Medicine/Bachelor of Surgery (MBBS), representing 86% of this cohort (Table 6.1). In total 64.5% of the 664 respondents were females, with 35.5% being males and no respondents identifying with any other gender categories. Of the total cohort, 67.5% were born in Australia and 32.5% overseas, with Singapore, Malaysia, New Zealand, India, Sri Lanka and China the most frequent responses, occurring 41, 24, 24, 21, 18 and 14 times respectively. Approximately 43% of the cohort was currently employed, working an average of

**Table 6.1**  Student demographic characteristics by degree

| Variables | HSC n (%) | BMS n (%) | MBBS n (%) | Total N (%) |
|---|---|---|---|---|
| Number of students | 114 (17.2) | 286 (43.1) | 264 (39.8) | 664 (100) |
| Age (yrs) | | | | |
| 18–21 | 108 (94.7) | 285 (99.7) | 263 (99.6) | 656 (98.8) |
| 22–30 | 5 (4.3) | 1 (0.3) | 1 (0.4) | 7 (1.1) |
| 31–40 | 1 (1.0) | 0 (0.0) | 0 (0.0) | 1 (0.1) |
| Gender | | | | |
| • Female | 93 (81.6) | 177 (61.9) | 158 (59.8) | 428 (64.5) |
| • Male | 21 (18.4) | 109 (38.1) | 106 (40.2) | 236 (35.5) |
| Ethnicity | | | | |
| • Australian born | 86 (75.4) | 197 (68.9) | 165 (62.5) | 448 (67.5) |
| • Born overseas | 28 (24.6) | 89 (31.1) | 99 (37.5) | 216 (32.5) |
| Currently employed | | | | |
| • Yes | 68 (59.6) | 139 (48.6) | 78 (29.5) | 287 (43.2) |
| • No | 46 (40.4) | 145 (50.6) | 184 (69.7) | 375 (56.5) |

12.5 hours per week, with individual responses ranging from one to 40 hours of paid employment per week.

In total, 96% of the student cohort reported watching television within the last year (Table 6.2). The four percent indicating that they did not watch television were from the BMS and MBBS degree programmes. When it came to regular television viewing choices, approximately 78% of the cohort reported watching comedies, 79% dramas, 92% movies, 71% news programmes, 52% sports, 55% documentaries and 62% regularly watching medical television shows.

When students were specifically asked about their watching preferences in terms of medical television shows, approximately 38% never watched medical television, whilst 48% reported occasional viewing and 14% reported frequent viewing. Students were not provided any guidelines for what constituted 'occasional' versus 'frequent' viewing, so were reporting the level of their engagement according to their own perception. In some cases, students who claimed to have 'never watched' medical dramas later in the questionnaire provided evidence that they were in fact engaging with these shows to some degree. In addition to the three main shows under consideration—*Grey's Anatomy, Scrubs* and *House, M.D.*—the other medical television shows that were watched most regularly included *Embarrassing Bodies, M\*A\*S\*H, Hart of Dixie, Private Practice, ER, R.P.A., 24 Hours in Emergency, King's Cross ER, One Born*

**Table 6.2**  Student television watching and behaviours by degree

| Variables | HSC, n = 114 (%) | BMS, n = 286 (%) | MBBS, n = 264 (%) | Total, N = 664 (%) |
|---|---|---|---|---|
| Has watched television in the past year | | | | |
| Yes | 114 (100.0) | 271 (94.8) | 253 (95.8) | 638 (96.1) |
| No | 0 (0.0) | 15 (5.2) | 11 (4.2) | 26 (3.9) |
| Regularly watches: | | | | |
| • Comedy | 90 (78.9) | 226 (79.0) | 198 (75.0) | 516 (77.7) |
| • Drama | 90 (78.9) | 220 (76.9) | 223 (84.5) | 524 (78.9) |
| • Movies | 104 (91.2) | 259 (90.6) | 144 (54.5) | 609 (91.7) |
| • News | 85 (74.6) | 211 (73.8) | 177 (67.0) | 475 (71.5) |
| • Sports | 50 (43.8) | 156 (54.5) | 140 (53.0) | 348 (52.4) |
| • Documentaries | 62 (54.4) | 162 (56.6) | 139 (52.6) | 364 (54.8) |
| • Medical television | 70 (61.4) | 170 (59.4) | 172 (65.2) | 412 (62.0) |
| Watches medical television* | | | | |
| • Frequently | 12 (10.5) | 38. (13.3) | 41. (15.5) | 91. (13.7) |
| • Occasionally | 58 (50.9) | 132 (46.2) | 131 (49.6) | 321. (48.3) |
| • Never | 44 (38.6) | 116 (40.6) | 91 (34.5) | 251 (37.8) |
| Medical television generates ethical discussion | | | | |
| • Yes—discussion self-initiated | 9 (7.9) | 40 (14.0) | 23 (8.7) | 72. (10.8) |
| • Yes—discussion initiated by others | 4 (3.5) | 7 (2.4) | 6 (2.3) | 17. (2.6) |
| • Yes—discussion initiated by self and others | 27 (23.7) | 50 (17.5) | 44 (16.7) | 121. (18.2) |
| • No | 32 (28.1) | 61 (21.3) | 89 (33.7) | 182 (27.4) |

*Frequency as determined by the students' own perception

*Every Minute, All Saints, Nip/Tuck* and *Offspring*. A further 66 shows were listed by students in this freeform section of the questionnaire, with each of these appearing between one and five times across the cohort.

Students were asked about their behaviours after watching the medical television shows and 210–representing 32% of the overall cohort of students—reported that they engaged in ethical discussions regarding the content of the shows with others. Approximately 11% reported initiating

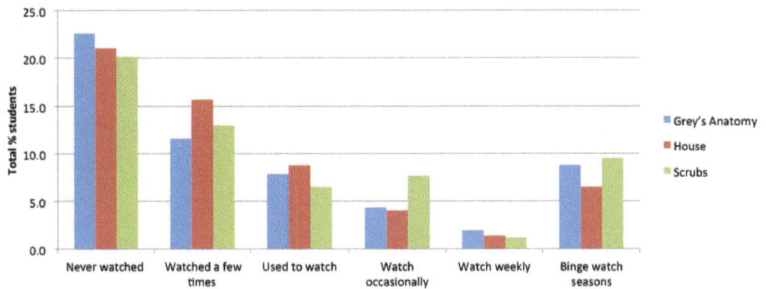

**Fig. 6.1**  Student television watching behaviours by show: *Grey's Anatomy, House, M.D.* and *Scrubs*

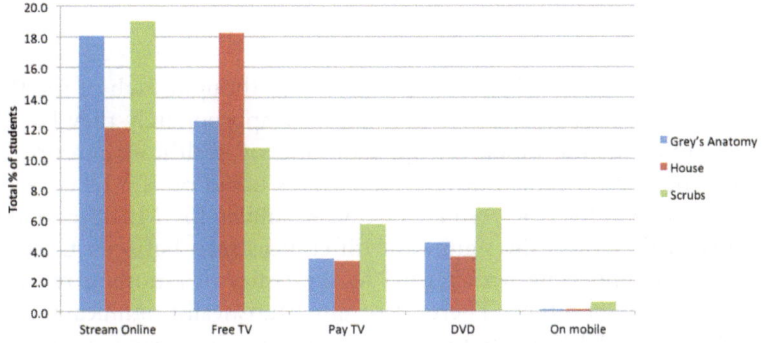

**Fig. 6.2**  Student television watching behaviours by method/source

these discussions themselves, 3% reported that others initiated these discussions with them and 18% reported that both they and others contributed equally to the ethical discussion.

Students were asked about their watching practices and behaviours in terms of medical television shows, paying particular attention to *Grey's Anatomy, Scrubs* and *House M.D.* (Fig. 6.1). A total of 229 students watched *Grey's Anatomy*, 251 students watched *Scrubs* and 241 watched *House M.D.* Streaming online and free television were the two most common watching methods (Fig. 6.2). Regarding their television viewing behaviours, 120, 128 and 159 students, respectively, watched the relevant television show with another person, whether family, friend, peer or colleague (Fig. 6.3).

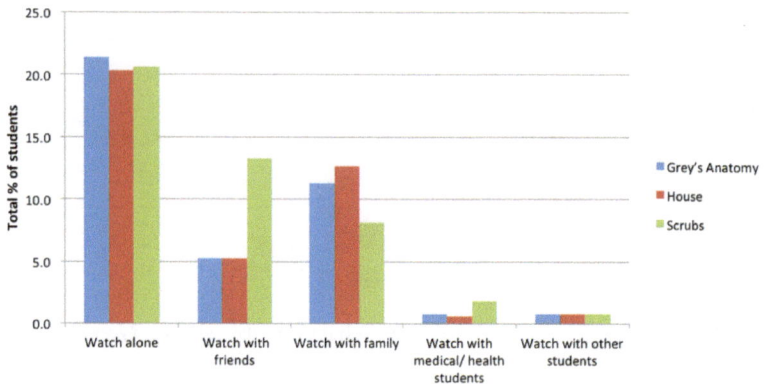

**Fig. 6.3**   Student television viewing behaviours

Students were also asked how accurate they thought each of the three major medical television shows was and how appropriately they handled certain ethical issues, ranging from rationing of healthcare resources to care for the dying (Table 6.3). Median scores based on the Likert scores were calculated, and the results were very similar for MBBS and BMS students, with statistically significant differences seen between these and the HSC students only with regard to the issues of rationing resources and medical misconduct. There were also statistically significant differences between MBBS students and the other two cohorts regarding the appropriateness of consent and confidentiality procedures in medical television shows. This is perhaps owing to less exposure to these issues in practice for these students, as they had less experience in the clinical setting, compared with the medical students. Regarding accuracy, HSC students rated *Grey's Anatomy* and *House, M.D.* higher than the BMS or MBBS students did, while the MBBS students found *Scrubs* the most accurate of the three.

Following the Likert scale questions there were a variety of free-form comments sections on the questionnaire, beginning with a question interrogating why students judged some medical television shows as depicting ethical and medical issues more accurately than others. While the total number of free-form responses was relatively low, it was still possible to observe certain patterns across the questions. That the show was marketed as a comedy was mentioned 46 times as a reason the show

**Table 6.3** Students' perceptions on accuracy and how appropriately issues are handled in medical television programmes

| | HSC | BMS | MBBS | p-value |
|---|---|---|---|---|
| *Television show's accuracy* | | | | |
| • *Grey's Anatomy* | 3.25 | 2.87 | 2.74 | 0.001 |
| • *House, M.D.* | 3.16 | 2.94 | 2.4 | <0.0001 |
| • *Scrubs* | 2.66 | 2.73 | 3.4 | <0.0001 |
| *Appropriate representation of issues* | | | | |
| Rationing resources | 3.3 | 2.9 | 2.8 | 0.0019 |
| Medical mistakes | 2.9 | 2.9 | 3.0 | 0.119 |
| Infectious diseases | 3.4 | 3.2 | 3.3 | 0.54 |
| Quality of life | 3.4 | 3.2 | 3.3 | 0.75 |
| Enhancement surgery | 3.0 | 3.0 | 2.9 | 0.16 |
| Medical education | 3.4 | 3.2 | 3.2 | 0.075 |
| Professional misconduct | 3.2 | 2.8 | 2.8 | 0.02 |
| Truth disclosure | 2.9 | 2.9 | 2.8 | 0.77 |
| Informed consent | 3.1 | 3.2 | 2.5 | <0.001 |
| Confidentiality | 3.1 | 3.0 | 2.7 | 0.025 |
| Access to healthcare | 3.3 | 3.1 | 3.1 | 0.14 |
| Human experiments | 3.1 | 2.8 | 2.9 | 0.14 |
| Organ/tissue transplants | 3.4 | 3.3 | 3.2 | 0.37 |
| Death and dying | 3.6 | 3.6 | 3.5 | 0.78 |

Likert score 5 = very accurate/appropriate, 4 = mostly accurate/appropriate, 3 = neutral, 4 = mostly inaccurate/inappropriate, 1 = very inaccurate/inappropriate

was less reliable, with a further 146 students claiming a show was 'less serious' if it was dramatic, comedic or romantic. There were 33 mentions of so-called 'medical documentary' shows, such as *R.P.A.* and *24 Hours in Emergency*, being more reliable as they were based on 'real' rather than fictional cases. Other reasons that students gave for whether they considered the shows to be accurate included how doctor–patient relationships were depicted (23 mentions) and how medical issues were presented (17). BMS and HSC students tended to rate *Scrubs* poorly in free-form comments, whereas several MBBS students reported being told by a lecturer in their course that this was one of the more accurate medical television shows, and thus they were more positive toward it. Twenty-eight students reported that television shows inappropriately exaggerated ethical dilemmas, with a further 20 saying important ethical issues were missing in the shows they watched.

When it came to which fictional characters from medical television shows students most wanted to be like, J.D. from *Scrubs* was the most popular choice, with 40 respondents selecting this character. This was followed by Dr House from *House M.D.* (33), Christina Yang from *Grey's Anatomy* (29) and Turk from *Scrubs* (25). When asked which characteristics made these role models attractive, being particularly talented or intelligent was the top choice with 56 mentions, which doubled the next most popular characteristic of being caring. Other top characteristics included being hard-working (22), compassionate (16), having a rewarding lifestyle (14) and behaving professionally (11). When asked the reciprocal question of which character they would least want to be like, Dr House received 44 votes, followed by Meredith Grey from *Grey's Anatomy* on 16 and Drs Kelso and Cox from *Scrubs* on 13 and 8, respectively. The top reasons supplied for these choices was that the character was selfish (12), uncaring (9), treated colleagues poorly (9), had an unpleasant life (9), behaved unethically (8) or was overconfident (8). There were also eight mentions that a character was overly emotional, annoying or 'whiny,' but these criticisms were exclusively directed at female characters.

When asked whether they recalled certain ideals of behaviour being depicted in medical television shows, and if so, whether these depictions were positive or negative, the overwhelming majority of respondents reported that the elements were present in the shows they watched and that they were treated positively (Fig. 6.4). The qualities of interest

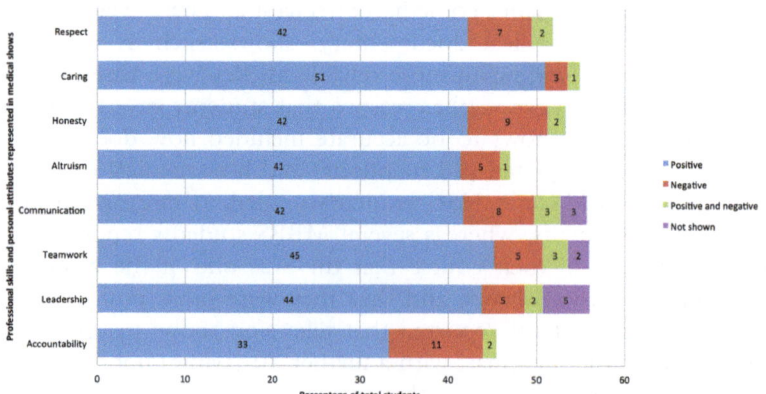

**Fig. 6.4**  Positive and negative representations of certain professional qualities and behaviours

**Table 6.4** Perceived influence of medical television shows on forming opinions

| Variables (n =# of respondents) | HSC | BMS | MBBS | p-value |
|---|---|---|---|---|
| Students' own opinions (n) | 102 | 266 | 248 | |
| Median likert score | 3.1 | 2.8 | 2.6 | 0.0005 |
| Students' thoughts on the opinions of family and friends (n) | 100 | 264 | 248 | |
| Median likert score | 3.3 | 2.9 | 3.1 | 0.069 |
| Students' thoughts on the opinions of policymakers (n) | 101 | 264 | 248 | |
| Median likert score | 2.9 | 2.5 | 2.3 | <0.0001 |

included personal traits, such as showing respect, being caring, honesty, and altruism, and professional skills, such as communication, teamwork, leadership, and accountability.

The final question on the questionnaire asked students how important they thought medical television shows were for forming opinions for themselves, their friends and family and policymakers (Table 6.4). HSC students reported much higher levels of influence for their own opinions than BMS or MBBS students. All three cohorts believed these shows were impacting the opinions of their friends and families but not policymakers, with MBBS students reporting the lowest perceived influence for this category.

## DISCUSSION

The results of the study indicate that HSC, BMS and MBBS students are high consumers of popular culture in the form of television, with over two-thirds engaging with medical television shows in particular. All three cohorts reported similar levels of exposure to most programme types, including medical television, with the only noteworthy difference being the reduction of MBBS students reporting watching movies, with approximately half of the medical student cohort selecting this option compared with over 90% in both of the other cohorts (see Table 6.2). While it is impossible to infer from the available data the reasons behind this difference, anecdotal evidence suggests medical students have less time to watch television so might prefer episodes, rather than full-length movies.

Students' preferred viewing methods were representative of the current delivery methods available, with online streaming services outstripping traditional viewing methods, such as DVD and free television in most cases. When it came to whether students watched medical television shows alone or with others, the majority of respondents reported solitary viewing. When students did watch these shows in company, *Grey's Anatomy* and *House, M.D.* were more likely to be watched with family, while *Scrubs* was most likely to be watched with friends, possibly owing to its comedic nature and the fact it is shorter than the other two (approximately 22 minutes per episode, compared with 44 minutes). While few students reported watching medical television on their mobile device, this may increase as a viewing method in the future as the technology progresses.

As anticipated, the three major shows—*Grey's Anatomy, House, M.D.*, and *Scrubs*—were the most frequently watched medical television shows by students in health-related degrees, currently or in the past. While at the time of reporting only *Grey's Anatomy* was still running, the enhanced availability of completed or cancelled television programmes on online streaming services is likely a contributing factor to their continued influence, particularly regarding the ability to 'binge' watch whole seasons of television on services such as Netflix. When comparing the frequency of medical television viewing for our cohort of medical students (65.2%) with that of the Weaver and Wilson study of 2011 (93.7%), the discontinuation of various, highly influential shows on prime-time television, including *ER*, *All Saints* and *Private Practice*, is a likely contributor to this outcome. Nevertheless, the results of the present study indicate that even shows that are considerably older, such as *M*A*S*H*, still possess cultural currency for students and thus could be used effectively in education. The presence of comments by MBBS students related to lecturers' positive opinions of *Scrubs*, coupled with the increased perception of accuracy of this show among this cohort compared with the others, is also telling in terms of the impact of educators' views on that of their students.

While most respondents were able to identify that there were a vast array of ethical issues present in the shows they watched, only one-third reported engaging in ethical discussions about these issues as a result of this exposure. When it came to how appropriately sensitive issues were handled on the shows, death and dying and organ and tissue transplants were perceived the best across all three cohorts, with medical mistakes, enhancement surgery, truth disclosure and human experimentation rated the most inappropriately handled overall. Regarding desirable personal traits and professional skills, all respondents reported seeing references to respect, caring, honesty and altruism in the shows they watched, but 2–5% claimed depictions of communication, teamwork and leadership skills were missing. According to the students, accountability was the element most likely to be negatively depicted in the fictional healthcare setting. While students were able to identify positive representations of ideal behaviours, the free-form comments seemed to betray a focus on intelligence or giftedness when selecting fictional role models, rather than caring attributes or appropriate behaviour.

Finally, students seemed unwilling to admit medical television shows might be influencing their own or policymakers' opinions in any way, but were more likely to consider their friends and family susceptible to its influence. This is particularly interesting in light of the research cited in earlier chapters, regarding the impact of medical television drama on medical students' practical skills—for example, for endotracheal intubation—and perceptions of best practice—for example, family presence during CPR.[9] The high response rate for the questionnaire, and the level of detail seen in some of the free-form comments, also indicates knowledge from these shows is being retained by students, whether they are aware of its influence or not. This provides further evidence that medical educators might have a vital role to play in mediating the knowledge being received through these sources.

## Strengths and Limitations

The major strengths of this study include the large sample size and the ability to directly compare the results with previous studies conducted under similar conditions using the pre-validated questionnaire. The extensive body of research available on the subject also helps paint a detailed picture of how medical students and those enrolled in other health-related degree programmes are engaging with popular culture representations of their chosen profession.

Regarding limitations, there is no follow-up component to this study, so changes cannot be tracked over time and it is not possible to establish a direct cause–effect relationship from this kind of study. For example, a student might express a certain opinion about the shows being assessed, but we are unable to establish from this study design whether their opinion was formed before or after exposure to the show itself. Individual students may change their opinions between their first and later years of study, but again we are unable to investigate this using a cross-sectional study design. Furthermore, while Likert scales are often considered to be a method of ascribing quantitative value to qualitative differences (e.g. the participant tries to estimate the magnitude of their opinion on a particular issue), they exist on a non-continuous scale, thereby limiting the statistical analyses possible.

Another potential limitation is that students who engaged with medical television were possibly more likely to complete the questionnaire than those who did not. As the questionnaires were conducted in class and the return rate was very high, it is believed that the effect of any difference in response rate was minimal. This may, however, account for the difference in exposure noted between our study and the two previous ones.

## CONCLUSION

Medical television dramas continue to entertain students in health-related degrees and the results of this study indicate there is the capacity to use these shows to educate students on medical and ethical issues as well. That students are able to identify ethical dilemmas in medical television shows but are less likely to initiate ethical debate on these topics, highlights an opportunity to bring these examples into the classroom to guide discussion and develop ethical reasoning skills for these future health professionals. This is expected to benefit students' learning, while also providing the skills required to engage future patients in medical and ethical discussions who might also be receiving health information from popular culture sources.

## NOTES

1. Bernard F. Lentz and David N. Laband, 'Why So Many Children of Doctors become Doctors: Nepotism vs. Human Capital Transfer,' *The Journal of Human Resources* 24, no. 3 (1989): 396–413.
2. Matthew J. Czarny, Ruth R. Faden, Marie T. Nolan, Edwin Bodensiek and Jeremy Sugarman, 'Medical and Nursing Students' Television Viewing Habits: Potential Implications for Bioethics,' *American Journal of Bioethics* 8, no. 12 (2008): 1–8.

3. Roslyn Weaver and Ian Wilson, 'Australian Medical Students' Perceptions of Professionalism and Ethics in Medical Television Programs,' *BMC Medical Education* 11 (2011): 50–5.
4. Brian Glasser, Michael Clark, Trisha Greenhalgh, Christine Harmar-Brown, Joan Leach, Michael Modell and John Salinsky, 'From Kafka to Casualty: Doctors and Medicine in Popular Culture and the Arts – A Special Studies Module,' *Medical Humanities* 27 (2001): 99–101.
5. Weaver and Wilson, 'Australian Medical Students,' 55.
6. Anna Pavlov and Gregory E. Dahlquist, 'Teaching Communication and Professionalism Using a Popular Medical Drama,' *Family Medicine* 42, no. 1 (2010): 25.
7. Gladys B. White, 'Capturing the Ethics Education Value of Television Medical Dramas,' *The American Journal of Bioethics* 8, no. 12 (2008): 14.
8. Weaver and Wilson, 'Australian Medical Students,' 50.
9. P.G. Brindley and C. Needham, 'Positioning Prior to Endotracheal Intubation on a Television Medical Drama: Perhaps Life Mimics Art,' [letter to the editor] *Resuscitation* 80 (2009): 604. For more detail on family presence during CPR please refer to Chap. 1 of this book.

**Acknowledgements** The authors would like to thank Roslyn Weaver and Ian Wilson for providing the template on which we built our questionnaire. We also wish to thank all the students who completed our study and the staff who facilitated this. Thanks are also due to Penelope J. Robinson, Divya Krishnan, Lenise Prater and Laura-Jane Maher who contributed to this research. This project was supported by the Monash University Faculty of Medicine, Nursing and Health Sciences, Learning and Teaching Research Grant Scheme and the Monash Education Academy, and was conducted for the Medical Education Research and Quality Unit (MERQ).

## Bibliography

Brindley, P.G. and C. Needham. 'Positioning Prior to Endotracheal Intubation on a Television Medical Drama: Perhaps Life Mimics Art.' [letter to the editor] *Resuscitation* 80 (2009): 604.

Czarny, Matthew J., Ruth R. Faden, Marie T. Nolan, Edwin Bodensiek and Jeremy Sugarman. 'Medical and Nursing Students' Television Viewing Habits: Potential Implications for Bioethics.' *American Journal of Bioethics* 8, no. 12 (2008): 1–8.

Glasser, Brian, Michael Clark, Trisha Greenhalgh, Christine Harmar-Brown, Joan Leach, Michael Modell and John Salinsky. 'From Kafka to Casualty: Doctors and Medicine in Popular Culture and the Arts – A Special Studies Module.' *Medical Humanities* 27 (2001): 99–101.

Lentz, Bernard F. and David N. Laband. 'Why So Many Children of Doctors become Doctors: Nepotism vs. Human Capital Transfer.' *The Journal of Human Resources* 24, no. 3 (1989): 396–413.

Pavlov, Anna and Gregory E. Dahlquist. 'Teaching Communication and Professionalism Using a Popular Medical Drama.' *Family Medicine* 42, no. 1 (2010): 25–7.

Weaver, Roslyn and Ian Wilson. 'Australian Medical Students' Perceptions of Professionalism and Ethics in Medical Television Programs.' *BMC Medical Education* 11 (2011): 50–5.

White, Gladys B. 'Capturing the Ethics Education Value of Television Medical Dramas.' *The American Journal of Bioethics* 8, no. 12 (2008): 13–4.

## CHAPTER 7

# Teaching Millennials: A Three-Year Review of the Use of Twitter in Undergraduate Health Education

## Basia Diug and Evie Kendal

The term 'Web 2.0' was first coined in 2004 and described a dramatic shift in how people interacted with online platforms and web-based information.[1] This primarily involved a move away from passive consumption to active, participatory creation of online content. A major contributor to this change was the rise of social media networking sites such as Facebook and Twitter. Each minute it is estimated that 695,000 Facebook status updates occur and 98,000 'tweets' are sent.[2] A tweet is a micro-blog limited to 140 characters, and unlike most Facebook pages, Scanfeld et al. note that the majority of Twitter accounts—94% as of August 2009—are public.[3] Twitter currently remains one of the fastest growing social media platforms,[4] and according to Robillard et al. is one of the top ten most visited websites on the internet with over 500 million global users.[5] Research on the use of social media in healthcare

B. Diug (✉) · E. Kendal
Monash University, Melbourne, VIC, Australia
e-mail: basia.diug@monash.edu

E. Kendal
e-mail: evie.kendal@monash.edu

© The Author(s) 2017
E. Kendal and B. Diug (eds.), *Teaching Medicine and Medical Ethics Using Popular Culture*, Palgrave Studies in Science and Popular Culture, DOI 10.1007/978-3-319-65451-5_7

indicates that Twitter is the most commonly used platform for disseminating public health information,[6] and has been used effectively when dealing with emergencies, such as natural disasters.[7]

Social media provides access to a vast online audience and offers the opportunity to engage various stakeholders involved in public health services and information provision. For Robillard et al. one of the major advantages of using social media to disseminate health knowledge is the fact that web and mobile-based applications 'reach a broad audience in a very short period of time, are easy and affordable to access and use, and cater for a wide variety of audiences.'[8] A study of the use of social media in health promotion in the United States indicated that local health departments predominantly used Twitter to 'inform, educate, and empower people' to make positive health choices.[9] A secondary use was as a complement or substitute for other disease surveillance mechanisms, owing to the unique advantage of providing geo-located data and trends in real-time (e.g. tracking the progress of a flu epidemic by mapping related social media posts). While it is less developed than its use in health promotion, Stoove and Pedrana claim the use of social media analysis in disease surveillance provides timely information, contributing to what has come to be known as the 'infoveillance' or 'infodemiology' of an outbreak.[10] Rather than relying on delayed data collection methods and self-reported questionnaires, this use of Twitter global positioning system (GPS) data allows for rapid location monitoring.[11] It also provides qualitative data regarding the population's attitudes and behaviours toward a health crisis or intervention and allows for wide-scale health communication.[12] This is particularly valuable in light of a 2009 Pew Research Center study that found 37% of American adults reported being influenced in their health-related decision-making by 'user-generated health information.'[13] This shift from seeking 'top-down' disclosure from health professionals and organisations, to peer-based user-created content as a source of health information has both positive and negative potential, as not all online health-related material is reliable or safe. This indicates a need to develop critical thinking skills among patients and health professionals who may be exposed to such information or hope to harness some of the power of social media in disseminating accurate health information.

The educational potential of Twitter is the primary focus of this chapter. The current cohort of tertiary students predominantly belongs to 'Generation Y,' a term used by demographers to refer to people born in the 1980s and 90s whose characteristics include high-level computer literacy.[14] Also known as 'digital natives' or 'millennials,'[15] this generation uses the internet as a primary communication method and source of useful information.[16] Sue Peattie notes this cohort are likely to respond better to health information they can access online, as they control their own exposure and level of engagement, as opposed to feeling like they are just being 'told what to do.'[17] As such, she claims internet-based public health campaigns are more empowering for the younger generation, as they provide the relevant health facts and then leave young people to make their own decisions. However, it is not just Generation Y who are seeking health information online, with a 2011 Pew Research Center survey in America indicating 80% of adult internet users now source health information on the web, a population including 85% of 50–64 year olds and 58% of over 65s.[18] When it comes to social media in particular, 15% of adult users directly report receiving health information from social media sources, with a further 23% following the personal health stories of their friends through these platforms.[19] A study by Stroever et al. looking at how well social media sources of health information were trusted by populations for whom traditional health communication methods were more difficult to achieve, indicated that if social media sites were run by 'university, government, or nonprofit organizations' this increased the perceived credibility of the information.[20] Given the potential to reach a vast audience and impact health behaviours, there is a clear need to train future health professionals on the most effective way to engage online audiences in health-related dialogue.

Our previous work investigated whether Twitter can, or should, be used as an educational tool.[21] This study indicated that in a structured format there are benefits to using Twitter-related activities in a tertiary curriculum, specifically in terms of enhancing access to staff and engagement with learning content. Therefore, we aimed to longitudinally evaluate the effectiveness of a Twitter-related assessment across a three-year period, and identify its effectiveness in increasing student engagement with public health concepts and facilitating staff and peer interactions.

## METHOD

In order to evaluate the benefit of exposing students of health-related disciplines to Twitter as a public health tool, a social media task was embedded as a graded assessment within a core first year public health unit in the Bachelor of Biomedical Science (BMS) degree at an Australian university. Students were given the choice of completing the assessment on a standard learning management system (Moodle) or using Twitter, and could further volunteer their data to be collected for this study if they chose (see Appendix). Participation involved the completion of a questionnaire after the end of semester regarding students' attitudes toward the social media task. This methodology was repeated on each of the first year BMS cohorts from 2014 to 2016.

The assessment consisted of six activities, with students instructed to tweet using the hashtag established for the unit so their contributions could be tracked:

1. Students were first instructed to download the app 'Dumb Ways to Die,' a game developed for Metro Trains in Victoria, Australia, as a public safety awareness campaign. The aim of the game is to survive as long as possible while engaging in a series of risky activities—for example, poking a grizzly bear with a stick—drawing analogies between these 'dumb' ways to die and being unsafe around trains. Students then tweeted their 'death,' final score and opinion of the game.

2. For the 'Public Health in Daily Life' challenge, students identified a public health issue in their everyday life and posted a photo or link to a newspaper or journal article about it. Examples included photos of hand sanitisers in hospital corridors, road safety signs and posters encouraging the use of stairs instead of lifts, to name a few. Students then had to explain their choice and why it was significant.

3. For the challenge entitled 'It's in the Media,' students posted on a public health issue they'd encountered in the media, including recent disease outbreaks, fad diet scandals, celebrity health promotion campaigns and so on. Students were encouraged to re-tweet assessments from trusted sources, such as the World Health Organization, or state health authorities.[22]

4. Following on from their experience identifying a relevant media article, students were next required to tweet the title and main findings of a peer-reviewed journal article on any health issue.

5. For the 'You Said, I Think' challenge, students had to comment on a peer's tweet, noting why they thought the topic chosen was

important. This was intended to increase collaboration across the student cohort.

6. Finally, students had to complete the 'I Can Do Better' challenge, in which they designed a health promotion campaign related to the topic of their media or journal article. They were required to write a brief overview of the strategy, target audience and method of dissemination.

Students who opted in to complete the research questionnaire were first asked to report their contributions, whether they engaged on Twitter more than the minimum required for the assessment and whether they had prior experience with social media, and if so, which platforms they used (Appendix: Student self-report). They were then asked to judge whether they thought the assessment task achieved its objectives, including promoting awareness of public health, whether they thought Twitter could support any other objectives in the education setting, and finally, whether they thought Twitter was an appropriate medium for this kind of assessment. Those students wishing to provide further feedback were asked to supply contact details for a follow-up focus group session.

All students had to complete an online professionalism agreement, with the 2016 cohort provided specific training in e-professionalism. This training outlined how to use social media in a professional and personal capacity, noted possible limitations regarding the use of Twitter as a professional tool, and detailed relevant behavioural and privacy matters. Students were moderated across all three years with any cases of unprofessional online conduct managed in line with university policies. Ethics approval for the study was provided by the Monash University Human Research Ethics Committee.

## Results

In total, 1303 out of 1447 eligible students completed the questionnaire across the three years, yielding an overall response rate of 90% (Table 7.1). As the cohort size increased each year, the proportion of students completing the Twitter-related activity and questionnaires also increased. In 2014, 332 students completed the questionnaire out of the 398 students enrolled in the unit, representing a response rate of approximately 83%. In 2015 this increased to 424 of the 466 enrolled students, a response rate of approximately 91%, and finally in 2016 this increased

**Table 7.1**  Cohort demographic characteristics across the three-year period 2014–2016

| n (total students) | 2014 n = 398 (%) | 2015 n = 466 (%) | 2016 n = 654 (%) |
|---|---|---|---|
| Completed | 332 (83.4) | 424 (91.0) | 583 (93.8) |
| Incomplete/did not complete | 66 (16.6) | 47 (10.1) | 36 (6.2) |
| **Gender** | | | |
| · Males | 172 (43.2) | 198 (42.5) | 221 (37.9) |
| · Females | 226 (56.8) | 268 (57.5) | 362 (62.1) |

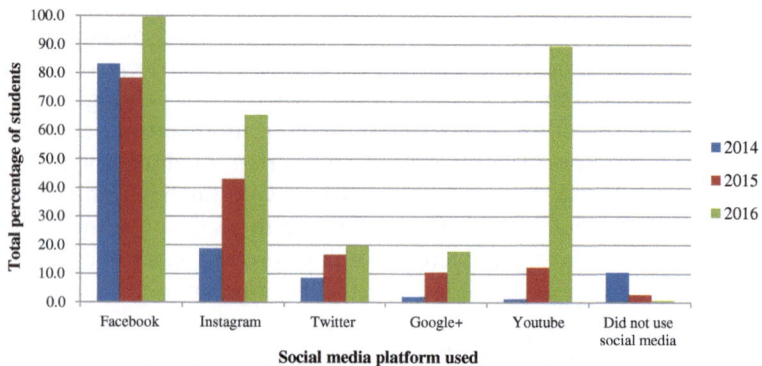

**Fig. 7.1**  Reported use of social media platforms prior to the study

to 547 of the 583 enrolled students, representing approximately 94% of this cohort. The gender split within the cohort was approximately 40% male and 60% female across the three years.

We compared across the three years the types of social media platforms that were utilised in this cohort (Fig. 7.1). During the three-year study period, Facebook remained the most popular social media platform used in the student cohort, with similar rates of adoption evident in 2014 and 2015, at 83 and 78% respectively. However, in 2016 there was a large jump in prior usage of Facebook to include almost the whole cohort, at 99.5%. Other significant changes in social media usage across this time period included the increased adoption of the photo-sharing app Instagram, with only 18.8% of the cohort reporting previous use of

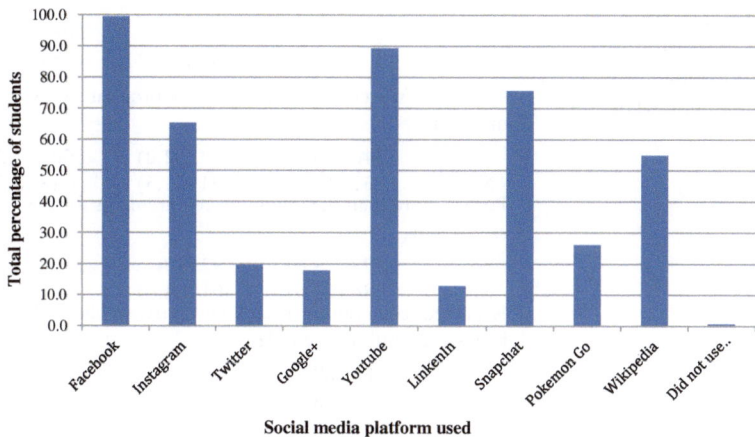

**Fig. 7.2** Comparison of prior use of social media and other online tools for BMS students in 2016

this platform in 2014, but 65.4% of respondents in 2016. Twitter also showed growth, doubling from 8.5 to 19.7% from 2014 to 2016. Use of the video-sharing platform YouTube demonstrated the most significant increase from 1.3 to 89.4% in 2016. Notably, those who did not use any social media decreased from 10.6% in 2014 to 0.7%—just four students—in 2016.

In 2016, additional data was gathered regarding other online tools and new social media platforms, including LinkedIn, Snapchat, Pokemon Go and Wikipedia (Fig. 7.2). Snapchat was the most popular, with 75.6% of the cohort using the 'self-destructing' photo- and video-sharing platform, whilst the global collaborative encyclopaedia website, Wikipedia, was used by 54.9%. The new Pokemon Go mobile app game was used by 26.1%, whilst only 12.9% used LinkedIn, the professional profile service.

Students were asked to appraise the Twitter-related activity for its appropriateness in the course (Table 7.2). In 2014, 86.9% found it appropriate for the assessment task, whilst in 2016, 90.2% of the cohort found it appropriate. In 2015 only 62.0% of the cohort found the task appropriate. Regarding whether students contributed and engaged more than the assessment task required, in 2014 almost 74.6% made additional posts, which decreased to 19.7% in 2015 and then increased again in 2016 to almost half the cohort. Across all three years, over 75% of

**Table 7.2** Student self-report thoughts on appropriateness and engagement across the three years

| Variables | 2014<br>n = 398 (%) | 2015<br>n = 466 (%) | 2016<br>n = 654 (%) |
|---|---|---|---|
| Consider Twitter-related activity an appropriate assessment medium | | | |
| · Yes | 346 (86.9) | 289 (62.0) | 550 (94.2) |
| · No | 52 (13.1) | 104 (24.5) | 48 (8.2) |
| Posted more than the minimum requirements for the assessment | | | |
| · Yes | 297 (74.6) | 92 (19.7) | 293 (44.8) |
| · No | 86 (21.6) | 301 (64.6) | 361 (55.2) |
| Reported feeling more aware of everyday public health issues as a result of the tasks | | | |
| · Yes | 356 (89.4) | 346 (74.1) | 51 (79.1) |
| · No | 22 (5.5) | 125 (26.8) | 75 (11.5) |

respondents felt that the Twitter-related task made them more aware of public health issues in their daily lives.

Regarding whether the activity impacted perceptions of staff accessibility, there was no significant difference between the three groups with mean scores of 2.1 (±SD 0.56) in 2014, 1.9 (±SD 0.66) in 2015 and 1.9 (±SD 0.73) in 2016, indicating that all three cohorts reported that the task made teaching staff more accessible (Fig. 7.3; Table 7.3).

When asked to self-report on how the Twitter-related activity impacted on their peer collaborations, there was again no significant difference between the three groups, with mean scores of 2.1 (±SD 0.53) in 2014, 2.3 (±SD 0.74) in 2015 and 2.3 (±SD 0.73) in 2016, indicating that all three cohorts agreed that the task had increased peer collaboration (Fig. 7.4; Table 7.4).

## DISCUSSION

Our findings highlight that students are vast consumers of social media and are willing to engage with social media platforms in the higher education setting. This is clearly seen in the response rate of 90% across the three cohorts. Further, our undergraduates have continued to be strongly engaged in social media platforms and are increasing the different types of platforms they are using, with 99.5% of the 2016 cohort using Facebook and 75.6% of that cohort using the newer platform Snapchat. The only reported decrease in the three years was the number

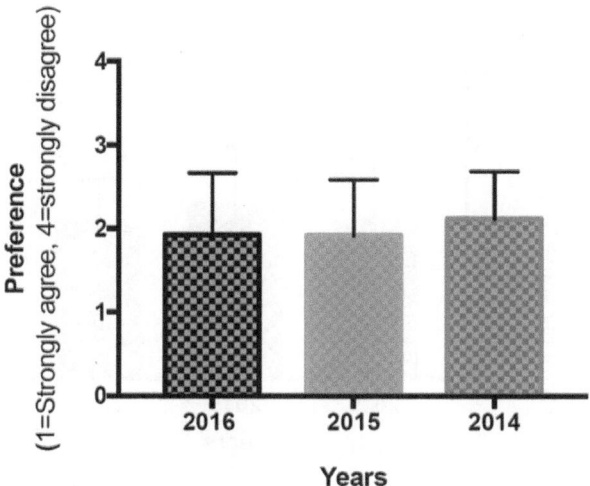

**Fig. 7.3** Students' perception of staff accessibility and Twitter-related assessment (Likert scales where strongly agree = 1, agree = 2, disagree = 3 and strongly disagree = 4)

**Table 7.3** Percentage of students' perception of staff accessibility

| Staff accessibility improved? | 2014 (%) | 2015 (%) | 2016 (%) |
| --- | --- | --- | --- |
| Strongly agree | 6.8 | 13.1 | 24.4 |
| Agree | 73.6 | 61.2 | 60.4 |
| Disagree | 10.8 | 6.9 | 9.1 |
| Strongly disagree | 3.5 | 3.2 | 4.8 |

of students who did not use social media. In general the vast majority of students found that using Twitter-related activities was appropriate in this context and reported that it increased their engagement with the course content. Overall, students also reported that this assessment increased their access to staff and peer collaboration across the three years.

In 2016, the Australian Sensis social media report was released. It confirmed our longitudinal three-year evaluation that the digital landscape continues to grow rapidly, with more than 87% of Australians

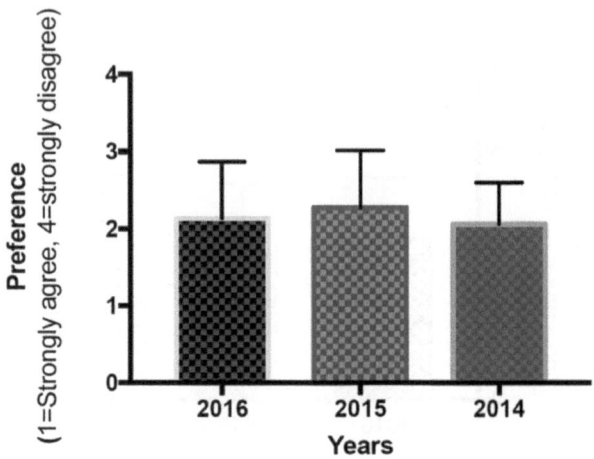

**Fig. 7.4** Students' perception of peer collaboration and Twitter-related assessment (Likert scales where strongly agree = 1, agree = 2, disagree = 3, and strongly disagree = 4)

**Table 7.4** Percentage of students' perception of peer collaboration

| Peer collaboration improved? | 2014 | 2015 | 2016 |
|---|---|---|---|
| Strongly agree | 10.6 | 8.6 | 15.6 |
| Agree | 69.3 | 50.6 | 59.2 |
| Disagree | 15.3 | 18.5 | 18.7 |
| Strongly disagree | 0.5 | 6.4 | 4.8 |

accessing the internet daily.[23] Of the social networking sites, Facebook remained the most used, with 95% of the study population using the platform, growing from previous years.[24] This is in keeping with our findings, with a decline in those who did not use social media and a steep increase over the three years of students using multiple social media platforms. The popularity of Snapchat across the Australian population was only 24%, compared to our cohort in which 75.6% used the platform. It was difficult to compare Snapchat in previous years as applications and networking sites are always changing in both popularity and usage. This is one of the key challenges when implementing and capturing the use of social media platforms in the classroom. Changes in student engagement in this domain are not necessarily consistent with population averages, owing to the higher proportion of younger people in the tertiary environment. Educators need to be aware that their choice of social media platforms requires clear scaffolding in the curriculum, with an understanding of the longevity and potential evolution of the platform. Our choice of the public health campaign app 'Dumb Ways to Die' bridged the gap between gamification and student learning outcomes. The application's popularity also paved the way for further engagement with gamification strategies in tertiary teaching, including the development of a card game for exam revision tutorials.

The assigned Twitter tasks were refined over the three years of the study, incorporating feedback from previous students about how best to integrate the activities into the unit to achieve the learning objectives. This involved repeated mentions of what was happening on Twitter in the lectures, tutorials and online discussion boards for the unit, embedding the Twitter feed for the unit's hashtag into the Moodle site and arranging for 'live tweeting' of lectures throughout the semester, including in one panel-style lecture fashioned in the style of the ABC television program, *Q&A*. In this lecture, students could 'live tweet' questions for the panel on a variety of pre-arranged topics, including the Belle Gibson celebrity diet scandal. Another refinement made to the Twitter assessment over the three years was increasing the number of challenges and the marks associated with the task from 2% of the students' final grade to 5%, which may account for some of the increase in completion rates between 2014 and 2016. It was consistent across the three years that student perceptions of increased staff accessibility and peer collaboration were a clear outcome of the Twitter-related activity.

Based on the questionnaire responses, most students welcomed the alternative assessment mode and felt it complemented the other, more traditional, assessment tasks in the unit. Most importantly, regarding the potential for Twitter to be used as a public health education tool, the majority of students reported this task made them feel more aware of public health issues. Whether this awareness will translate into greater uptake of Twitter and other social media platforms for their future work in public health education and promotion is yet to be seen, but it is hoped this early exposure will have an impact in this area. Furthermore, the additional training in e-professionalism is expected to have long-lasting benefits for millennial students, who are the first generation to grow up with social media profiles. In a 2010 interview for *The Wall*

*Street Journal,* then Google CEO Eric Schmidt claimed that lack of awareness among young people of the extended reach and long-term impact of social media use would leave many seeking name changes later in life, particularly when attempting to enter the workforce.[25] Coupled with the potential impact of using social media in health communication discussed at the beginning of this chapter, this supports the idea that university educators can fulfil a much-needed role for students within the health and medical fields, by exposing them to the power of social media as a public health tool and training them how to use this tool in a professional manner.

One of the most important outcomes of this project was the need to train students in e-professionalism and appropriate online behaviour in the educational setting. After some concerns regarding unprofessional behaviour, an e-book resource was developed for students that outlined how employability and future opportunities could be impacted by a poor online presence or 'brand.' This resource was then embedded into the curriculum of both this unit and others at the university. Since then, no instances of inappropriate behaviour have been observed and reported. Nevertheless, this experience highlighted the need for close monitoring of online engagements related to curricula, even when such engagements are typically public, as in the case of social media posts.

The key strengths of this study include the longitudinal nature and the large sample size of participants. This is further supported by the 90% response rate and task completion over the three years. However, limitations of this study include limited prior exposure of the cohort to Twitter, and the need to develop clear e-professionalism training, which was only discovered part-way through the project. These risk management areas are requirements when using an open access application such as Twitter with a student cohort. Further, despite the implication that these students are 'digital natives,' it is necessary to support them when using a new application so that they can benefit from this interaction.

## Conclusion

The use of social media is part of our everyday lives and therefore also in the lives of our student cohort. Increased uptake of social media platforms, including Twitter and Facebook, amongst our students is a reality that has the potential to be translated and utilised as a positive educational tool. Despite the rapid uptake, we need to ensure that our cohorts are guided to use these platforms in a structured manner that can support the development of key graduate attributes. E-professionalism that focuses online conduct is at the heart of our student development and is a necessity for any task that uses these platforms. Our longitudinal study found that students self-reported increased engagement with the unit content, increased accessibility to staff and an increase in peer collaboration as a result of the use of social media in the classroom. Additional research is required to evaluate whether this assessment has an impact on learning and student grades.

## NOTES

1. Daniel Scanfeld, Vanessa Scanfeld and Elaine L. Larson, 'Dissemination of Health Information Through Social Networks: Twitter and Antibiotics,' *American Journal of Infection Control* 38, no. 3 (2010): 182.
2. Jeff Tieman, 'The Facebook Frontier: Compelling Social Media Can Transform Health Dialogue,' *Health Progress* 93, no. 2 (2012): 82.
3. Scanfeld et al. 'Dissemination of Health Information,' 183.
4. Mary Lou Manning and James Davis, 'Journal Club: Twitter as a Source of Vaccination Information: Content Drivers and What They're Saying,' *American Journal of Infection Control* 41 (2013): 571.
5. Julie M. Robillard, Thomas W. Johnson, Craig Hennessey, B. Lynn Beattie and Judy Illes, 'Aging 2.0: Health Information about Dementia on Twitter,' *PLoS One* 8, no. 7 (2013): e69861, DOI:10.1371.
6. Brad L. Neiger, Rosemary Thackeray, Scott H. Burton, Callie R. Thackeray and Jennifer H. Reese, 'Use of Twitter Among Local Health Departments: An Analysis of Information Sharing, Engagement, and Action,' *Journal of Medical Internet Research* 15, no. 8 (2013): e177.
7. Robillard et al. 'Aging 2.0.'
8. Ibid.
9. Neiger et al. 'Use of Twitter.'
10. Mark A. Stoove and Alisa E. Pedrana, 'Making the Most of a Brave New World: Opportunities and Considerations for Using Twitter as a Public Health Monitoring Tool,' *Preventive Medicine* 63 (2014): 109.
11. Scott H. Burton, Kesler W. Tanner, Christophe G. Giraud-Carrier, Joshua H. West and Michael D. Barnes, '"Right Time, Right Place" Health Communication on Twitter: Value and Accuracy of Location Information,' *Journal of Medical Internet Research* 14, no. 6 (2012): e156.
12. Ibid.
13. Scanfeld et al. 'Dissemination of Health Information,'186.

14. Sue Peattie, 'Using the Internet to Communicate the Sun-safety Message to Teenagers,' *Health Education* 102, no. 5 (2002): 212.
15. Pew Research Center, 'Millennials in Adulthood: Detached from Institutions, Networked with Friends' (7 March 2014). Available at: http://www.pewsocialtrends.org/2014/03/07/millennials-in-adulthood/.
16. Peattie, 'Using the Internet,' 212.
17. Ibid., 216.
18. Robillard et al. 'Aging 2.0.'
19. Susannah Fox, 'The Social Life of Health Information, 2011,' Pew Research Center (12 May 2011). Available at: http://www.pewinternet.org/files/old-media/Files/Reports/2011/PIP_Social_Life_of_Health_Info.pdf; Jenine K. Harris, Nancy L. Mueller, Doneisha Snider and Debra Haire-Joshu, 'Local Health Department Use of Twitter to Disseminate Diabetes Information, United States,' *Preventing Chronic Disease* 10 (2013): 120215.
20. Stephanie J. Stroever, Michael S. Mackert, Alfred L. McAlister and Deanna M. Hoelscher, 'Using Social Media to Communicate Child Health Information to Low-income Parents,' *Preventing Chronic Disease* 8, no. 6 (2011): A148.
21. Basia Diug, Evie Kendal and Dragan Ilic, 'Evaluating the Use of Twitter as a Tool to Increase Engagement in Medical Education,' *Education for Health* 29, no. 3 (2016).
22. These first three challenges made up the pilot version of this study, as reported above.
23. Sensis Social Media Report, 'How Australian People are Using Social Media' (2016). Available at: https://www.sensis.com.au/asset/PDFdirectory/Sensis_Social_Media_Report_2016.PDF, 7.
24. Ibid., 4.
25. Holman W. Jenkins, Jnr, 'The Weekend Interview with Eric Schmidt: Google and the Search for the Future,' *The Wall Street Journal*, New York, 4 August 2010.

APPENDIX: QUESTIONNAIRE
ASSESSMENT TASK: STUDENT SELF REPORT

1. Prior to this activity, did you use any online tools/social media? If so, select all that apply:
   (a) No, I don't use social media
   (b) Facebook
   (c) Instagram

(d) Twitter
(e) Google+
(f) LinkedIn
(g) Snapchat
(h) Pokemon Go
(i) YouTube
(j) Wikipedia

2. Do you think it was appropriate to use Twitter to complete this assessment task?
   (a) Yes
   (b) No

3. If No, why not?

4. Do you think the online participation task improved accessibility to staff? Pick only one answer:

| 1 | 2 | 3 | 4 |
|---|---|---|---|
| Strongly agree | Agree | Disagree | Strongly disagree |

5. Did you find the weekly posts from the staff helpful?

6. Do you think the online participation task promoted collaboration with peers? Pick only one answer:

| 1 | 2 | 3 | 4 |
|---|---|---|---|
| Strongly agree | Agree | Disagree | Strongly disagree |

7. During semester did you post more than required for the online participation task? If yes, please estimate how many times?

8. True or False: I feel this activity positively influenced my educational experience:
   (a) True
   (b) False

9. True or False: I feel that the Twitter activity made me MORE aware of public health in our daily lives:
   (a) True
   (b) False

10. True or False: I found the Twitter feed on Moodle a good way to see what other students are posting and engage with them:
    (a) True
    (b) False

11. True or False: I found the Twitter activity in the tutorial a good
way to see what other students are posting and engage with them:
(a) True
(b) False

## BIBLIOGRAPHY

Burton, Scott H., Kesler W. Tanner, Christophe G. Giraud-Carrier, Joshua
H. West and Michael D. Barnes. '"Right Time, Right Place" Health
Communication on Twitter: Value and Accuracy of Location Information.'
*Journal of Medical Internet Research* 14, no. 6 (2012): e156.

Diug, Basia, Evie Kendal and Dragan Ilic. 'Evaluating the Use of Twitter as a
Tool to Increase Engagement in Medical Education.' *Education for Health*
29, no. 3 (2016).

Fox, Susannah. 'The Social Life of Health Information, 2011.' Pew Research
Center (12 May 2011). Available at: http://www.pewinternet.org/files/old-
media/Files/Reports/2011/PIP_Social_Life_of_Health_Info.pdf.

Harris, Jenine K., Nancy L. Mueller, Doneisha Snider and Debra Haire-
Joshu. 'Local Health Department Use of Twitter to Disseminate Diabetes
Information, United States.' *Preventing Chronic Disease* 10 (2013): 120215.

Jenkins, Jnr., Holman W. 'The Weekend Interview with Eric Schmidt: Google
and the Search for the Future.' *The Wall Street Journal*, New York, 4 August,
2010.

Manning, Mary Lou and James Davis. 'Journal Club: Twitter as a Source
of Vaccination Information: Content Drivers and What They're Saying.'
*American Journal of Infection Control* 41 (2013): 571–572.

Neiger, Brad L., Rosemary Thackeray, Scott H. Burton, Callie R. Thackeray
and Jennifer H. Reese. 'Use of Twitter Among Local Health Departments:
An Analysis of Information Sharing, Engagement, and Action.' *Journal of
Medical Internet Research* 15, no. 8 (2013): e177.

Peattie, Sue. 'Using the Internet to Communicate the Sun-safety Message to
Teenagers.' *Health Education* 102, no. 5 (2002): 210–218.

Pew Research Center. 'Millennials in Adulthood: Detached from Institutions,
Networked with Friends.' (7 March 2014), available at: http://www.pewso-
cialtrends.org/2014/03/07/Millennials-in-adulthood/.

Robillard, Julie M., Thomas W. Johnson, Craig Hennessey, B. Lynn Beattie and
Judy Illes. 'Aging 2.0: Health Information about Dementia on Twitter.' *PLoS
One* 8, no. 7 (2013): e69861, DOI:10.1371.

Scanfeld, Daniel, Vanessa Scanfeld and Elaine L. Larson. 'Dissemination of
Health Information Through Social Networks: Twitter and Antibiotics.'
*American Journal of Infection Control* 38, no. 3 (2010): 182–188.

Sensis Social Media Report. 'How Australian People are Using Social Media.' (2016). Available at: https://www.sensis.com.au/asset/PDFdirectory/Sensis_Social_Media_Report_2016.PDF.

Stoove, Mark A. and Alisa E. Pedrana. 'Making the Most of a Brave New World: Opportunities and Considerations for Using Twitter as a Public Health Monitoring Tool.' *Preventive Medicine* 63 (2014): 109–111.

Stroever, Stephanie J., Michael S. Mackert, Alfred L. McAlister and Deanna M. Hoelscher. 'Using Social Media to Communicate Child Health Information to Low-income Parents.' *Preventing Chronic Disease* 8, no. 6 (2011): A148.

Tieman, Jeff. 'The Facebook Frontier: Compelling Social Media Can Transform Health Dialogue.' *Health Progress* 93, no. 2 (2012): 82–83.

# Balancing the Needs of the Many Against the Needs of the Few: Aliens, Holograms and Discussions of Medical Ethics

*Allie Ford and Lynette Pretorius*

Healthcare educators need to prepare their students to become effective medical professionals, capable of utilising their own personal wisdom as well as several different ethical theories and codes of conduct in their practice. This involves providing training so that students can be professionally socialised and gain an understanding of appropriate ethical behaviour in their discipline.[1] However, medical ethics is a challenging concept to teach, as it is complex, cognitively demanding and often subjective. Pedagogic innovation can therefore be beneficial in creating learning opportunities that allow students to explore medical ethics and their own social and cultural biases in an experiential way.

A. Ford (✉) · L. Pretorius
Monash University, Melbourne, VIC, Australia
e-mail: allie.ford@monash.edu

L. Pretorius
e-mail: lynette.pretorius@monash.edu

© The Author(s) 2017                                                              133
E. Kendal and B. Diug (eds.), *Teaching Medicine and Medical Ethics Using Popular Culture*, Palgrave Studies in Science and Popular Culture,
DOI 10.1007/978-3-319-65451-5_8

Throughout history science fiction has provided a literary vehicle to explore science, technology, philosophy and society's visions of the future. One of the largest science fiction phenomena to date is the *Star Trek* franchise. The first *Star Trek* television series (entitled *Star Trek*, now referred to as *Star Trek: The Original Series*) was aired between 1966 and 1969. In subsequent years, four additional television series were released: *Star Trek: The Next Generation* (1987–94), *Star Trek: Deep Space Nine* (1993–9), *Star Trek: Voyager* (1995–2001) and *Star Trek: Enterprise* (2001–5). Thirteen motion pictures have also been released (1979–2016).

Previous research has shown that complex social, moral or ethical problems can be approached in a more open-minded manner if they are presented in a fictional context. For example, Joyce Fields showed that the complex concept of sociological imagination (an awareness of the interrelated nature of one's personal experience and the wider society) could be taught in an introductory sociology subject using *Harry Potter*.[2] The *Star Trek* universe similarly provides an effective literary vehicle to examine ethical and moral questions associated with modern science and technology. A previous study showed that the *Star Trek: The Next Generation* episode *Ethics* could be used at a first-year level,[3] to teach students about medical ethics and the doctor–patient relationship.[4] The scripts of *Star Trek* are presented as modern philosophical parables.[4] An important feature of the vast *Star Trek* universe is that it contains hundreds of unknown species, each with their own cultures and beliefs.[4] It has been argued that within one series, or even within one episode, ethical philosophies can vary dramatically between individuals, creating an environment without a single overarching moral code.[4,5] This fictional setting therefore allows discussions that are free from traditional societal or cultural biases, since people are less likely to have a pre-conceived bias about an alien species compared with a particular human race or culture.[4,5] Furthermore, each episode is usually self-contained, so a detailed understanding of the franchise or the particular *Star Trek* series is not required for effective teaching.

Many episodes of *Star Trek* incorporate ethical dilemmas in healthcare and can therefore be useful teaching resources to introduce students to the concepts of medical ethics. In this chapter we will focus on two episodes from *Star Trek: Voyager*: *Nothing Human* (Season 5, Episode 8),[6] and *Critical Care* (Season 7, Episode 5).[7] We have chosen these episodes as they can be used in conjunction with each other to examine all four of the key principles of medical ethics (respect for autonomy, non-maleficence, beneficence and justice).[8] Furthermore, both episodes are effective in highlighting a situation where the ship's doctor decides to compromise his own moral code in order to fully meet the needs of his patients. In the following sections we describe how each of these episodes can be used as an effective teaching strategy to evoke deeper learning and improve student engagement.

## EXPLORING THE PRINCIPLES OF MEDICAL ETHICS USING STAR TREK

A key figure in the *Star Trek* universe is the Science Officer from *The Original Series*—a Vulcan commander named Spock. In *Star Trek*, Vulcans are known for their attempts to make decisions based only on logic, without interference from emotion.[9] One of the most well-known Vulcan ethical philosophies is the need to benefit the greatest number of individuals, even at the expense of sacrificing the interests or well-being of a few. This philosophy permeates the *Star Trek* universe and demonstrates a consequentialist morality. Consequentialism advocates for the greatest good for the greatest number and evaluates morality based on the consequences of an action.[8] In a very real sense this philosophy also permeates healthcare settings. For example, consequentialist ideals are relevant in hospital triage settings, where healthcare staff need to determine where their time and resources would be of greatest benefit to the largest number of patients. Furthermore, the treatment of individual patients also incorporates consequentialist considerations by highlighting that the greatest good is the action that best fulfils the preferences of the patient.[8] Students are therefore likely to face consequentialist considerations throughout their medical practice.

An effective way to introduce consequentialist considerations to new students is to consider the use of unethically obtained research to treat patients effectively. It is a common misconception among new students that they will not encounter this ethical concern in their practice. It is important to challenge this perception, however, as several medical breakthroughs, even relatively recently, were indeed developed as a result of unethically conducted research. Consider, for example, the HeLa cell line found in most laboratories worldwide. This immortal cell line was created from tissue obtained from a terminally ill patient named

Henrietta Lacks.[10,11] Importantly, this tissue was obtained without the knowledge or consent of the patient or her family, largely owing to racial and economic prejudice at the time.[10] HeLa cells are currently the most commonly used human cell line in scientific research and are used to study biochemical processes in healthy and diseased tissue.[11,12] These cells have been used to produce treatments for various medical conditions including polio, cancer, influenza, haemophilia and Parkinson's disease.[10,11] By 2013 it was estimated that over 70,000 scientific articles had been published based on the HeLa cell line.[12] It is therefore very likely that students will at some point in their future practice interact with a treatment discovered or developed using HeLa cells.

The *Star Trek*: Voyager episode *Nothing Human* examines issues surrounding the use of unethically obtained research.[6] In particular it focuses on the use of medical research obtained through wartime atrocities. The episode's exploration of this issue relates to all four key principles of medical ethics, making it a useful teaching resource, particularly at the beginning of ethical training for pre-service clinicians. There are also clear parallels in this episode to the unethical medical research conducted by Nazi doctors during the Second World War that involved murder, torture and several other atrocities.[13] This episode is therefore particularly useful in highlighting the relevance of this topic to modern medicine.

Experiential learning, which allows students to create meaning for themselves through self-discovery, involves four stages: concrete experience, reflective observation, abstract conceptualisation and active experimentation.[14] Experiential learning is most effective when it involves a reflective learning phase, a time of deeper learning where students represent their learning and a time for learning from feedback.[15] Consequently, we suggest that educators use the *Star Trek* episode as a pre-class activity, requiring students to watch the episode in its entirety before class. This will allow students to experience the story through individual exploration, helping them to evaluate and reflect on their own personal views.

In order to allow students to present their learning in a reflective manner, it is suggested that each learner completes a reflective journal after watching the episode. The benefits of reflective journaling have been well documented, particularly in encouraging students to reflect on their experiences.[16,17] Research has also shown that reflective practice allows medical professionals to discover personal beliefs and attitudes, become more self-aware and ultimately improve their practice.[18–20] Furthermore, reflective practice allows the identification of educational needs, engaging professionals in the process of life-long learning.[20,21] We have previously described a template for reflection (based on Gary Rolfe's minimal model of reflective practice),[22] which allowed students to focus on their experiences rather than academic content.[23] We suggest a similar journal template should be used for this learning experience.

For students to gain genuine knowledge from the experience, educators also need to provide engaging activities during class time to build upon the pre-class activity. We have described some of these activities later in this chapter. These activities incorporate peer discussion and feedback, allowing students to contextualise the experience and apply it to their future practice.

## Synopsis and Dramatis Personae of Star Trek: Voyager

*Star Trek*: Voyager is set in the twenty-fourth century and follows the adventures of the crew of the starship Voyager as they attempt to return home from the distant Delta Quadrant, where they were stranded during their inaugural mission.[24] The episodes described below are set in seasons five and seven of the series and include the following key characters: Captain Kathryn Janeway (Captain of Voyager), Commander Chakotay (First Officer), Lieutenant Commander Tuvok (Security/Tactical Officer), Lieutenant B'Elanna Torres (Chief Engineer), Lieutenant Tom Paris (Helmsman), Ensign Harry Kim (Operations Officer), the Emergency Medical Hologram known as the Doctor (Chief Medical Officer) and Seven of Nine (known colloquially as 'Seven,' Astrometrics Crewman).[24] Most of these crew members are human, with the exception of Lieutenant Commander Tuvok (Vulcan), Lieutenant Torres (Half Human/Half Klingon, a warrior race that primarily values honour),[25] and the Doctor (a computer program). Seven is human but was captured as a child by the Borg, a cybernetic life form with a collective consciousness that incorporates other species into its collective through cybernetic assimilation.[26] She was liberated from the Borg but still retains some cybernetic implants.

## STAR TREK: VOYAGER: NOTHING HUMAN

The crew of Voyager encounter a distress call from an injured alien life form and decide to provide assistance. While the Doctor attempts to diagnose and cure his alien patient, the injured life form attaches itself to the ship's Chief Engineer—Lieutenant Torres. As the Doctor tries to detach the life form, he realises that it has attached itself to Lieutenant Torres' vital organs and that removal would likely result in the death of both his patients.

In consideration of the Doctor's lack of expertise in exobiology, Captain Janeway asks Ensign Kim to create a holographic consultant to help treat Lieutenant Torres. The Doctor decides to base the hologram on a well-known expert in the field named Crell Moset. The Doctor and Moset quickly start working on a potential treatment and in the process develop a professional friendship. However, it is soon discovered that Moset derived his expertise from wartime atrocities during which he murdered hundreds in the pursuit of medical progress, including the family of one of the junior crew members of the ship (Ensign Tabor).

The ensign tells the Doctor how Moset killed his grandfather during radiation experiments, as well as blinding and burning others to investigate their healing and adaptation processes. The Doctor is initially sceptical, noting that Moset was responsible for curing an epidemic. The Ensign is unimpressed, noting that the cost of this cure was borne by the many others who had been the subjects of Moset's experiments. The Doctor continues to resist blaming Moset, pointing out that there are no entries about his activities in the Enterprise computer. Commander Chakotay points out that those using questionable practices do not often publicise their actions. Nevertheless, the Doctor remains doubtful; Moset now holds a prestigious position at a respected university.

Despite the fact that Moset appears to be Lieutenant Torres' only hope for a cure, she refuses to accept any further treatment based on his wartime research. The rest of the episode centres on whether it is appropriate to use Moset's expertise. Ultimately, Captain Janeway decides to overrule Lieutenant Torres' objections and allow the Doctor to use Moset's treatment. The Doctor and Moset proceed with the treatment and manage to separate the life form and Lieutenant Torres. Both patients survive and the life form is returned to other members of its species. After the procedure, however, Lieutenant Torres is very upset that she was treated against her wishes.

After consideration, the Doctor decides to delete Moset's program and all its unethically acquired knowledge from the ship's computer. In the last scene of the episode, the Doctor informs Moset of his decision. Their ensuing discussion highlights the complexities surrounding the use of unethically obtained research when a patient's life lies in the balance. As they talk, Moset is triumphant about their joint success in saving both patients. When the Doctor questions the source of that success, Moset's wartime research, Moset instead questions the Doctor's own willingness to use that same research when his patient's life hung in the balance. The conversation, rather than providing clear-cut judgement on the moral issues highlighted in the episode, challenges each viewer to reach their own conclusions.

## Learning Activities

As noted above, it is necessary to supplement self-discovery learning experiences with classroom activities that provide students with a time to represent their learning and a time to learn from feedback. In order to achieve this, we suggest that class time following this pre-class activity can be broadly divided into three sections: reflections from the experience, contextualising the experience and applying the experience to future practice. Learning activities for each of these sections are described below. These activities will allow students to develop a basic and personal understanding of each of the key principles of medical ethics.

## Reflections from the Experience

At the start of the class, students should be asked to identify the ethical or moral issues highlighted in the episode, using their reflective journals if required. In consideration of the established benefits of shared learning, we suggest that this activity would be best conducted in small groups of three to four students. Following small group discussion, a larger group discussion should be facilitated by the teacher to collect the reflections from each small group. This part of the class should be designed to allow students to categorise their identified issues into overarching ethical theme clusters. Through in-depth group discussion, this activity can be used to highlight all four key medical ethics principles.

## CONTEXTUALISING THE EXPERIENCE

The second part of the class should contextualise the learning experience. In order to achieve this, we suggest providing the following activity to students and allowing small group and larger group discussion.

> A central ethical principle in the *Star Trek* universe is the importance of balancing the needs of individuals against the requirements and rights of larger groups. However, in this episode, Captain Janeway decides to allow the Doctor to use the unethically obtained wartime research to cure his patient, despite the fact that many people suffered or died in the pursuit of this research. This can be considered as placing the needs of the few (the individual patient) over the needs of the many (the people who suffered or died in the wartime experiments). Do you think it is more important to prioritise the needs of the many, or is it more important to ensure that the needs of the individual patient are met? Why?

## APPLYING THE EXPERIENCE TO FUTURE PRACTICE

The final part of the class is designed to allow students to apply what they have learned to future clinical practice. In order to achieve this, students should be provided with the following small-group discussion prompt.

> In the *Star Trek* episode you watched, Moset claims that the Doctor's argument for terminating his holographic program, based on Moset's wartime research activities, is unjustified, because the Doctor was prepared to use the results of that research.
>
> Their conversation highlights the complexities of deciding whether to use unethically obtained research, particularly when a patient's life lies in the balance. In current clinical practice, healthcare professionals are also faced with deciding whether to use unethically obtained research.
>
> Consider the case of Henrietta Lacks we have provided. Do you think the actions of the doctor who first obtained the HeLa cells were justified? Despite now knowing how the HeLa cells were

> obtained, scientific research still continues to use these cells. Is this justified? Why or why not?

## Encouraging Deeper Learning Through the Establishment of a Learning Community

In order to encourage deeper learning, we recommend that a second learning experience using the *Star Trek*: Voyager episode *Critical Care* should be incorporated into students' medical ethics training.[7] This episode further explores the concepts of justice, beneficence and non-maleficence in clinical practice, with a particular focus on the just allocation of medical resources. Research has demonstrated that participation in a learning community increases student engagement.[27] We believe that allowing students to collectively bear witness to the experiences of the Doctor will foster the development of a learning community, so we recommend that this episode should be watched together in class.

## *Star Trek*: Voyager: *Critical Care*

The Doctor's program is activated in what appears to be a medical facility by a man who wants to sell him to the hospital administrator (Chellick). Realising that he has been stolen from Voyager, the Doctor initially refuses to work for his kidnappers. However, when he is confronted with a large number of trauma victims, the Doctor decides that the patients' need for his help outweighs his moral objections.

As the Doctor starts treating the patients, he discovers that the hospital is poorly staffed and lacks basic equipment and medicine. Additionally, he finds that he is not able to treat his patients effectively because they have low 'TC' scores. Before the Doctor is able to discover what a TC is, however, the hospital administrator transfers him to Level Blue where he is told his services are most needed. The Doctor assumes that Level Blue is the critical care area, and Chellick agrees that it is the place where quality care is most required.

At this point we recommend the video should be paused and students asked to identify what they would expect to find in the Level Blue area. Following group discussion, the video should be resumed. The Doctor discovers that Level Blue is in fact a vastly better resourced section of the hospital with only a few patients, none of whom appear to need critical care. He soon discovers that these patients are receiving preferential treatment because their TC is higher than other patients. When he investigates further, the Doctor discovers that TC is a treatment coefficient, a value assigned to each patient upon their arrival at the hospital by a computer program called the Allocator. The TC is determined by a person's current and projected future worth to society. As a result of this system, the Allocator assigns higher TCs to wealthy, famous or important members of society, while socially inferior patients are denied life-saving care. Chellick notes that the algorithm is necessary in order to balance the level of care provided with the hospital's available resources.

As the Doctor starts treating the patients in Level Blue, he discovers that they are prescribed medicine for non-life saving treatments that are designed to increase life expectancy. This includes using daily injections of the medicine desperately needed in the other area of the hospital. The Doctor is confronted with the injustice of this system, and decides to try and circumvent the established protocols to make the system less discriminatory. He steals medication from Level Blue and uses it to treat several patients on Level Red (where those with lower TC scores are treated). Unfortunately, the Doctor's actions are soon discovered, leading to many critically ill patients being discharged because they have exceeded their permitted allocation of treatment for the year. This means that all the patients the Doctor treated are likely to die.

The hospital administrator decides to restrict the Doctor to Level Blue and gives the Allocator the power to override the Doctor's program. The Doctor, however, enlists the help of a staff member from the other part of the hospital and returns to Level Red. When he is discovered, the administrator decides it is time to deactivate the Doctor's program, but is not able to do so before the Doctor injects the administrator with the same virus that has caused so much suffering on Level Red. Explaining the injection to a Level Red physician, the Doctor explains that he is experimenting with a new treatment to improve empathy—in Chellick's case by changing his role (and perspective) from hospital administrator to patient. The Doctor also tricks the Allocator into thinking the administrator's TC is lower than it should be, so he is denied access to the cure. The Doctor uses Chellick's desire for the medicine as leverage to provide the medication to all Level Red patients who need it. Their conversation highlights the different priorities of their roles: the Doctor is focussed on preserving life, while the administrator is more concerned about the well-being of the wealthy patients who presumably fund the hospital.

When the Doctor is rescued by his shipmates, he partially regrets his actions and expresses a hope that his decision to threaten the administrator with death was caused by a malfunction in his system. After a diagnostic, however, the Doctor is informed that his ethical subroutines are working perfectly—he cannot use them to explain his actions. Seven of Nine, who ran the diagnostic, identifies that the Doctor's actions make perfect sense in Borg ideology; he put the well-being of the collective ahead of that of a specific individual. The Doctor notes that he is not happy with this comparison to the Borg (who are well known within the *Star Trek* universe for their focus on subsuming all individuals and species they meet into their collective—with or without consent).[26]

## LEARNING ACTIVITIES

A key threshold concept in medical ethics is the realisation that there is not always a right or wrong answer in clinical practice. Learning activities that evoke an understanding of this threshold concept will result in deeper learning. We propose that the following two activities will allow students to foster their own understanding of the complexities of medical ethics. First, the following discussion prompt can be used to stimulate classroom discussion about whether the Doctor acted ethically in this episode.

> The Doctor asks Seven to do a diagnostic of the ethical aspects of his program because he thinks it was a malfunction in his system that allowed him to poison the hospital administrator, acting against his imperative, as a Doctor, to do no harm. However, after the diagnostic the Doctor discovers there was no malfunction and that his ethical subroutines are in fact working perfectly. Are the Doctor's actions therefore justifiable? Why or why not?

Secondly, we recommend that this learning experience should be complemented by the following reflective activity to promote self-discovery and personal growth. Since this is likely to be a challenging task, we recommend that students should be told that their reflections will remain private and that they will not be required to submit them after class.

> 1. In this episode the Doctor decides that the needs of the many terminally ill patients on Level Red are most important, so he reallocates medicine that was intended for Level Blue patients. Identify at least one ethical reason why this action can be justified and one reason why this action could be considered unethical.
> 2. When the Doctor's actions are discovered, all the patients he treated with the stolen medicine are sent home because they have exceeded their annual allotment of medication. It is likely all of these patients will die. Write a reflective journal entry, examining how you feel about the Doctor's actions. Do you think he made the right decision? Why or why not? What would you have done differently?

## CONCLUSION

Educators can explore real-world ethical issues in the fictional universe of *Star Trek*. In this chapter we have demonstrated a strategy for teaching the key principles of medical ethics using two episodes from *Star Trek: Voyager*. A similar strategy can also be effective in many other disciplines in higher education, as the *Star Trek* universe addresses ethical and moral dilemmas in a variety of spheres including philosophy, anthropology, sociology, artificial intelligence, law and religion. We therefore suggest that *Star Trek* can be used as an interdisciplinary literary vehicle to encourage students to engage effectively with technical content in a fictional environment.

## NOTES

1. J. Summers, 'Theory of Healthcare Ethics,' in *Health Care Ethics: Critical Issues for the 21st Century*, 3rd ed., Eds. E.E. Morrison and B. Furlong (Burlington, MA: Jones & Bartlett Learning, 2014), 3–45.
2. J.W. Fields, 'Harry Potter, Benjamin Bloom, and the Sociological Imagination,' *International Journal of Teaching and Learning in Higher Education* 19, no. 2 (2007): 167–77.

3. C. Chalmers, 'Ethics,' *Star Trek: The Next Generation*, Season 5, Episode 16, Screened 29 February 1992 (United States of America: Paramount Pictures, 1992).
4. J.J. Hughes, and J.D. Lantos, 'Medical Ethics through the Star Trek Lens,' *Literature and Medicine* 20, no. 1 (2001): 26–38.
5. J.A. Barad, *The Ethics of Star Trek* (New York: Perennial, 2001).
6. D. Livingston, 'Nothing Human,' *Star Trek: Voyager*, Season 5, Episode 8, screened 2 December 1998 (United States of America: United Paramount Network, 1998). Television Broadcast.
7. T. Windell, 'Critical Care,' *Star Trek: Voyager*, Season 7, Episode 5, screened 1 November 2000 (United States of America: United Paramount Network, 2000). Television Broadcast.
8. T.L. Beauchamp and J.F. Childress, *Principles of Biomedical Ethics*, 7th ed. (New York: Oxford University Press, 2012).
9. 'Vulcans,' *Star Trek Database*, accessed 28 June 2016, available at: http://www.startrek.com/database_article/vulcans.
10. R. Skloot, *The Immortal Life of Henrietta Lacks* (Sydney: Pan Macmillan, 2010).
11. J.R. Masters, 'Hela Cells 50 Years On: The Good, the Bad and the Ugly,' *Nature Reviews Cancer* 2, no. 4 (2002): 315–19.
12. J.J.M. Landry, P.T. Pyl, T. Rausch, T. Zichner, M.M. Tekkedil, A.M. Stütz et al. 'The Genomic and Transcriptomic Landscape of a Hela Cell Line,' *G3: Genes|Genomes|Genetics* 3, no. 8 (2013): 1213–24.
13. The Nuremberg Trials Project. *Medical Case Transcript*, Harvard Law School Library Digital Document Collection, available at: http://nuremberg.law.harvard.edu/.
14. D.A. Kolb, *Experiential Learning: Experience as the Source of Learning and Development* (Englewood Cliffs, NJ: Prentice Hall, 1984).
15. J. Moon, *A Handbook of Reflective and Experiential Learning: Theory and Practice* (London: Routledge Falmer, 2004).
16. S. Epp, 'The Value of Reflective Journaling in Undergraduate Nursing Education: A Literature Review,' *International Journal of Nursing Studies* 45, no. 9 (2008): 1379–88.
17. D.D. Stevens and J.E. Cooper, *Journal Keeping: How to Use Reflective Writing for Learning, Teaching, Professional Insight, and Positive Change* (Sterling, VA: Stylus, 2009).
18. A. Bandura, *Social Foundations of Thought and Action: A Social Cognitive Theory* (Englewood Cliffs, NJ: Prentice Hall, 1986).
19. R.M. Epstein, 'Mindful Practice,' *Journal of the American Medical Association* 282, no. 9 (1999): 833–9.
20. K. Mann, J. Gordon, and A. MacLeod, 'Reflection and Reflective Practice in Health Professions Education: A Systematic Review,' *Advances*

*in Health Sciences Education: Theory and Practice* 14, no. 4 (2009): 595–621.

21. D. Boud, R. Keogh and D. Walker, *Reflection: Turning Experience into Learning* (London: Kogan Page, 1985).
22. G. Rolfe, D. Freshwater and M. Jasper, *Critical Reflection for Nursing and the Helping Professions: A User's Guide* (Basingstoke: Palgrave Macmillan, 2001).
23. L. Pretorius and A. Ford, 'Reflection for Learning: Teaching Reflective Practice at the Beginning of University Study,' *International Journal of Teaching and Learning in Higher Education* 28, no. 2 (2016): 241–52.
24. Star Trek: Voyager,' Star Trek Database, accessed 28 June 2016, available at: http://www.startrek.com/page/star-trek-voyager.
25. 'Klingons,' Star Trek Database, accessed 28 June 2016, available at: http://www.startrek.com/database_article/klingons.
26. 'Borg,' Star Trek Database, accessed 28 June 2016, available at: http://www.startrek.com/database_article/borg.
27. L.M. Rocconi, 'The Impact of Learning Communities on First Year Students' Growth and Development in College,' *Research in Higher Education* 52, no. 2 (2011): 178–93.

**Acknowledgements**  *Star Trek* is a trademark of CBS Studios Inc.

## BIBLIOGRAPHY

Bandura, A. *Social Foundations of Thought and Action: A Social Cognitive Theory.* Englewood Cliffs, NJ: Prentice Hall, 1986.
Barad, J.A. *The Ethics of Star Trek.* New York: Perennial, 2001.
Beauchamp, T.L. and J.F. Childress. *Principles of Biomedical Ethics,* 7th ed. New York: Oxford University Press, 2012.
Boud, D., R. Keogh and D. Walker. *Reflection: Turning Experience into Learning,* London: Kogan Page, 1985.
Chalmers, C. 'Ethics,' *Star Trek: The Next Generation,* Season 5, Episode 16, Screened 29 February 1992. United States of America: Paramount Pictures, 1992.
Epp, S. 'The Value of Reflective Journaling in Undergraduate Nursing Education: A Literature Review.' *International Journal of Nursing Studies* 45, no. 9 (2008): 1379–88.
Epstein, R.M. 'Mindful Practice.' *Journal of the Medical Association* 282, no. 9 (1999): 833–9.
Fields, J.W. 'Harry Potter, Benjamin Bloom, and the Sociological Imagination.' *International Journal of Teaching and Learning in Higher Education* 19, no. 2 (2007): 167–77.

Hughes, J.J. and J.D. Lantos. 'Medical Ethics through the Lens.' *Literature and Medicine* 20, no. 1 (2001): 26–38.

Kolb, D.A. *Experiential Learning: Experience as the Source of Learning and Development*. Englewood Cliffs, NJ: Prentice Hall, 1984.

Landry, J.J.M., P.T. Pyl, T. Rausch, T. Zichner, M.M. Tekkedil, A.M. Stütz et al. 'The Genomic and Transcriptomic Landscape of a Hela Cell Line.' *G3: Genes|Genomes|Genetics* 3, no. 8 (2013): 1213–24.

Livingston, D. 'Nothing Human,' *Star Trek: Voyager*, Season 5, Episode 8, screened 2 December 1998. United States of America: United Paramount Network, 1998.

Mann, K., J. Gordon and A. MacLeod. 'Reflection and Reflective Practice in Health Professions Education: A Systematic Review.' *Advances in Health Sciences Education: Theory and Practice* 14, no. 4 (2009): 595–621.

Masters, J.R. 'Hela Cells 50 Years On: The Good, the Bad and the Ugly.' *Nature Reviews Cancer* 2, no. 4 (2002): 315–19.

Meyer, N. *Star Trek II: The Wrath of Khan*, screened 4 June 1982. United States of America: Paramount Pictures, 1982.

Moon, J. *A Handbook of Reflective and Experiential Learning: Theory and Practice*. London: Routledge Falmer, 2004.

Morrison, E.E. and B. Furlong, . eds. *Health Care Ethics: Critical Issues for the 21st Century*, 3rd ed. Burlington, MA: Jones & Bartlett Learning, 2014.

Pretorius, L. and A. Ford. 'Reflection for Learning: Teaching Reflective Practice at the Beginning of University Study.' *International Journal of Teaching and Learning in Higher Education* 28, no. 2 (2016): 241–53.

Rocconi, L.M. 'The Impact of Learning Communities on First Year Students' Growth and Development in College.' *Research in Higher Education*, 52, no. 2 (2011): 178–93.

Rolfe, G., D. Freshwater and M. Jasper. *Critical Reflection for Nursing and the Helping Professions: A User's Guide*. Basingstoke: Palgrave Macmillan, 2001.

Skloot, R. *The Immortal Life of Henrietta Lacks*. Sydney: Pan Macmillan, 2010.

*Star Trek Database*. Accessed 28 June 2016, available at: http://www.startrek.com/database.

Stevens, D.D., and J.E. Cooper. *Journal Keeping: How to Use Reflective Writing for Learning, Teaching, Professional Insight, and Positive Change*. Sterling, VA: Stylus, 2009.

The Nuremberg Trials Project. *Medical Case Transcript*, Harvard Law School Library Digital Document Collection, available at: http://nuremberg.law.harvard.edu/.

Windell, T. 'Critical Care,' *Star Trek: Voyager*, Season 7, Episode 5, screened 1 November 2000. United States of America: United Paramount Network, 2000.

## CHAPTER 9

# Mind-Melds and Other Tricky Business: Teaching Threshold Concepts in Mental Health Preservice Training

*Lynette Pretorius and Allie Ford*

The incidence of diagnosed mental and behavioural disorders is increasing worldwide, contributing approximately 11% to the global burden of disease.[1] In Australia, these disorders affect approximately 7.3 million people at some point in their lifetime, contributing significantly to morbidity and mortality.[2] It is therefore becoming increasingly important for contemporary healthcare practitioners, regardless of their speciality, to be equipped with the skills necessary to work effectively and ethically with people experiencing mental illness.

The stereotyping of individuals with mental illness is widespread in society.[3] These stereotypes contribute to systemic negative attitudes towards mental illness and have arisen largely owing to fear and misunderstanding.[4] In modern society these negative stereotypes are often reinforced by inaccurate portrayals of mental illness in the media.[5] In

L. Pretorius (✉) · A. Ford
Monash University, Melbourne, VIC, Australia
e-mail: lynette.pretorius@monash.edu

A. Ford
e-mail: allie.ford@monash.edu

© The Author(s) 2017                                                             149
E. Kendal and B. Diug (eds.), *Teaching Medicine and Medical Ethics Using Popular Culture*, Palgrave Studies in Science and Popular Culture,
DOI 10.1007/978-3-319-65451-5_9

recent years mental health literacy has increased, particularly in relation to a more biological aetiology of disease.[6] However, many public attitudes towards people with mental illness have not changed, and in some cases have even worsened, particularly in relation to notions of dangerous behaviour.[6]

Research has shown that challenging inaccurate stereotypes through education can be successful in replacing judgements based on stereotypes with discernment grounded in factual information.[7] Furthermore, increased interpersonal contact between the public and a stigmatised group lessens prejudice.[7] Considering that most mental health professionals have received training and come into frequent contact with patients experiencing mental health challenges, it might be reasonable to expect that these practitioners have a greater awareness of the challenges faced by those with mental illness. However, Lauber and colleagues showed that the negative stereotyping of mental illness is perpetuated by both the general public and mental health professionals, particularly with respect to the 'dangerous' nature of those experiencing mental ill health.[3] This is concerning, and highlights that healthcare practitioners' actions and decisions are not only shaped by experiences and training, but also by personal and social stereotypes and biases, which can lead to attribution errors.[8,9]

## THRESHOLD CONCEPTS IN MENTAL HEALTH

In any subject there are a number of key topics, providing knowledge and skills appropriate to the area of study. Some of these concepts are gatekeepers to deeper knowledge, understanding and thinking in the discipline. Meyer and Land identify the latter as *threshold concepts* that allow students to genuinely see new perspectives and think in different ways.[10,11] Threshold concepts might be understood as 'lightbulb' moments, where illumination provides a new perspective leading to a permanent transformation of thought. This permanent change is one of the factors that distinguish threshold concepts from general content. Threshold concepts are therefore likely to be transformative, irreversible, integrative and troublesome.[11] Several barriers hinder or prevent students from crossing such thresholds; these barriers include conflicting knowledge that is traditional, ritualised, rarely used (such as unconnected or abstract ideas), conceptually difficult or counterintuitive, arising from different social, cultural or temporal norms, or where the holder of the knowledge is unaware of its existence.[11,12] Each of these barriers can play a significant role in preventing trainee healthcare professionals from developing a deep, personal and connected understanding of medical ethics until they enter professional practice.

Tanner identified several issues that practitioners classified as transformative or difficult in practice education.[13] For the purposes of this chapter we will focus on two of Tanner's areas of transformation: recognising personal and societal biases leading to fear and stigma associated with mental illness and realising the person with the mental illness is primarily a person.[13] We propose that these two transformative areas are threshold concepts that are necessary for students to develop an understanding of the larger concept of person-centred practice. The conceptual boundary of person-centred practice in mental health provision lies at the point of accepting that some stereotypes are incorrect or damaging. In particular, mental healthcare practitioners need to be able to see their patients as people first, not just as a diagnosis. This necessitates recognising and acknowledging any personal fears and prejudices relating to mental illness or people experiencing mental illness. This new understanding transforms the student, leading to a shift in thoughts, feelings and actions.

Some people experiencing mental illnesses can, at times, present with violent tendencies or confronting behaviours, providing additional challenges for mental health caregivers. This can be especially problematic for novice practitioners who may not previously have observed patients exhibiting similar behaviour. Pre-service training typically focuses on theoretical discussions of ethics using traditional teaching methods such as lectures, workshops, problem-based tasks, essays or case studies. These approaches are often directed towards traditional patients with physiological conditions, and can be effective in developing an academic understanding of ethical issues in healthcare provision. However, they do not necessarily encourage students to explore, reflect or engage with the complex nature of mental illness and its associated ethical challenges on a personal level. It is this deeper exploration that can prompt students to examine their own pre-suppositions or biases, leading to personal transformation. It is only by allowing students the time and space for their own lightbulb moments that they are able to illuminate new details or regions of their internal landscape of knowledge and understanding. It would therefore be of benefit to design learning experiences where students can experience, at least to an extent, situations where patients behave in a manner that conflicts with societal norms. Supportive visualisation of these situations through narrative and storytelling allows transformative learning in a low-risk environment.

In the rest of this chapter we will discuss how two stories from *Star Trek: Voyager* can be used to encourage exploration of the threshold concept of person-centred practice in a mental illness context. Literature has demonstrated that complex social, moral or ethical problems can be addressed in a learning environment when they are contextualised in the science fiction universe of *Star Trek*.[14,15] For example,[14] Hughes and Lantos showed that the *Star Trek: The Next Generation* episode *Ethics* could be effectively used to teach new students about medical ethics and the doctor–patient relationship.[16] In Chap. 8,[15] it was demonstrated that two episodes from *Star Trek: Voyager* could be effectively utilised to teach students about the four key principles of medical ethics (respect for autonomy, non-maleficence, beneficence and justice).[17] Several episodes in the *Star Trek* universe incorporate mental health considerations and are useful teaching resources in higher education settings. In this chapter we will focus on two episodes of *Star Trek: Voyager:* 'Meld' (Season 2, Episode 16),[18] and 'Death Wish' (Season 2, Episode 18).[19] We have chosen these episodes as they provide students with opportunities to observe behaviours or ideas that conflict with societal norms—violence and murder ('Meld') and suicide ('Death Wish'). Both episodes are effective in highlighting the complex nature of these behaviours, as well as the responses these behaviours elicit from others.

## Synopsis and Dramatis Personae of *Star Trek: Voyager*

*Star Trek: Voyager* is set in the twenty-fourth century and follows the adventures of the crew of the starship Voyager as they attempt to return home from the distant Delta Quadrant, where they were stranded during their inaugural mission.[20] The episodes 'Meld' and 'Death Wish' described below are set in season two of the series and include the following key characters: Captain Kathryn Janeway (Captain of Voyager), Lieutenant Tuvok (Security/Tactical Officer), Ensign Lon Suder (Engineer), the Emergency Medical Hologram known as the Doctor (Chief Medical Officer), Neelix (Morale Officer) and Kes (Medical Assistant).[20] The episode 'Death Wish' also incorporates two additional characters (Q and Quinn),[19] who are members of the Q Continuum, a species of immortal and seemingly omnipotent beings.[21] While the name

'Q' is used both collectively for the species, and individually by all members of the Q Continuum, one of the two Q adopts the name Quinn at the end of the episode. For purposes of clarity this name will be used to differentiate between the two characters.

## VIOLENCE AND MURDER

The *Star Trek: Voyager* episode 'Meld'[18] is a futuristic depiction of the effects of violent thoughts on the behaviours of two contrasting protagonists. Lieutenant Tuvok is a Vulcan, an alien species known for their attempts to make decisions based only on logic, without interference from emotion.[22] In contrast, Ensign Suder is a Betazoid (a telepathic and empathetic alien species),[23] who experiences extremely violent tendencies. Interestingly, the characteristics of these two protagonists switch halfway through the episode. This provides an excellent learning opportunity for students to examine how mental illness can change a person's behaviour. It also allows teachers to highlight that anyone can be affected by mental illness, allowing students to develop an understanding of the person behind the symptoms or behaviours.

Prior to class we suggest students should complete a personal reflective activity, examining their own biases about mental illness. The completion of a survey similar to the one described by Lauber and colleagues would be effective,[3] as it would allow students the opportunity to identify both the positive and negative stereotypes they associate with people experiencing mental illness. It would be beneficial to administer this activity anonymously and electronically as this will enable students to respond more freely, and allow the educator to collate the results for further discussion during class time. We recommend that the class should start with a screening of the episode, allowing students to collectively bear witness to the experiences of Lieutenant Tuvok and Ensign Suder.

## STAR TREK: VOYAGER: 'MELD'[18]

At the start of this episode, a murdered crewman is found in the Engineering section of the ship. The security officer, Lieutenant Tuvok, is called to investigate. Computer access logs and DNA evidence quickly demonstrate that only one person could be responsible for the crewman's death: Ensign Suder. When confronted with the evidence, Ensign

Suder confesses coldly and dispassionately, providing the details of the murder, but no clear motive.

The logic-focused Lieutenant Tuvok struggles to accept the fact that there is no obvious reason to explain the murder. He discusses Ensign Suder's mental state with the Doctor, hoping the actions can be explained by a psychotic illness. The Doctor, however, notes that most people have violent urges at times, and that many individuals or species learn to suppress them. He suggests that perhaps the murder was a result of a momentary lack of control, rather than any premeditation.

Not convinced by the Doctor's ideas, Lieutenant Tuvok decides to re-interview Ensign Suder, attempting to establish a motive by suggesting multiple logical explanations. However, Ensign Suder rejects each of these explanations. Being a Vulcan, Lieutenant Tuvok suggests that he would like to attempt a mind-meld (a telepathic technique that allows a Vulcan to merge their mind with the essence of another),[24] to better understand the Ensign's thoughts.

Suder is not convinced that the meld would be safe—for either of the participants. Tuvok counters his concerns by noting that as a Vulcan he has the ability to suppress any emotions spilling over from the meld, and that Suder will probably gain emotional regulation abilities, at least temporarily. Eventually they decide to proceed with the mind-meld.

Initially it does indeed seems to have benefited both participants. Lieutenant Tuvok confirms that there really was no significant motive for the murder and that it was the outcome of Suder's attempts to restrain his intrinsically violent temperament in a society where outlets for expressing such emotions are limited or non-existent. The mind-meld also leads to Ensign Suder gaining improved control over his emotions, allowing him to feel more centred and mindful of his emotions, especially his inner violent feelings, without letting them overwhelm him.

As the episode progresses, despite his earlier assurances that he had the skill to contain any feelings transferred from Suder during the meld, Lieutenant Tuvok begins to experience the residual violent tendencies from the mind-meld. When we next see him, he is approached by the Morale Officer, Neelix, in the dining area of the ship. Neelix attempts to coax Lieutenant Tuvok to smile, but the Vulcan responds explosively, strangling him. As Neelix lies dead on the floor, Lieutenant Tuvok asks the ship's computer to turn off the holodeck (a virtual reality environment where scenarios can be created and enacted holographically).[25] The audience learns that Lieutenant Tuvok has created this holographic scenario as a potential way to release violent impulses in a safe environment. During discussions with Ensign Suder about this technique, however, Lieutenant Tuvok realises he has indeed lost control of the residual feelings from the mind-meld, and that despite his earlier confidence he genuinely lacks the ability to suppress these violent instincts. In order to ensure the safety of the ship's crew, he locks himself in his living quarters, deactivates all his security clearances and informs Captain Janeway that he is unfit for duty.

Upon entering Lieutenant Tuvok's quarters, Captain Janeway finds that the normally logical and emotionally controlled Vulcan has destroyed his living quarters and is sitting in the dark. The Captain tries to convince him to go with her to get medical attention, but he advises her to stay away. Tuvok explains that his attempts at using traditional meditation techniques to control his feelings have failed; instead he has been fixating on identifying and counting the many different ways he knows of to kill people, using his extensive knowledge of martial arts.

Eventually, Captain Janeway convinces Lieutenant Tuvok to go to Sickbay by agreeing to sedate him in order to minimise the threat to the rest of the crew. The Doctor and his assistant, Kes, determine that Lieutenant Tuvok's abilities to suppress undesired emotions have been reduced. The medical team start the recommended treatment, which involves temporarily completely removing Lieutenant Tuvok's ability to control his emotions. This treatment is designed to function like an emotional defibrillator, resetting his neurological system and allowing his own processes to reassert themselves. The first treatment takes approximately three minutes, but during this time Lieutenant Tuvok becomes increasingly angry, arrogant, threatening and violent. As the treatment ends, he loses consciousness and is sedated. The Doctor tells the Captain that he does not know how much treatment will be required, or even if the treatment will ultimately provide a cure.

That evening Lieutenant Tuvok awakes in Sickbay, and while no one is around he manages to break through the force field designed to restrict his movements. He goes directly to the brig, intent on executing Ensign Suder for his crime. Suder challenges Tuvok to consider his actions; Tuvok focuses on the need for justice, but Suder suggests that perhaps he is actually looking to release his own emotions, or even seeking revenge. Suder explains that killing someone is a one-way street with no way back.

Lieutenant Tuvok attempts to forcefully initiate a mind-meld, but is unable to complete his actions, collapsing unconscious on the floor. Ensign Suder calls for medical assistance and Lieutenant Tuvok is transported back to Sickbay for further treatment. The Doctor, while reassuring Tuvok that his own emotional regulation systems did appear to be functioning, does question how healthy total emotional suppression is, in any species.

## LEARNING ACTIVITIES

Learning activities associated with the episode 'Meld' should allow students to explore, reflect on and engage with the threshold concepts that contribute to ethical person-centred practice in mental health-care provision: recognising personal and societal biases leading to fear and stigma associated with mental illness and realising the person with the mental illness is first and foremost a person. In particular, students should be given the opportunity to examine the strengths and weaknesses of their own ethical landscape and to apply this knowledge to future practice.

After screening the episode, students should be given time for individual private reflection to promote self-discovery and personal growth. This can be done using the reflective prompt below.

> Prior to attending today's class, you completed an online questionnaire about attitudes associated with mental illness.
>
> – Identify at least one attitude you had about people experiencing mental illness.
> – After watching the *Star Trek: Voyager* episode 'Meld,' has this attitude changed? What prompted the change, or reinforced your existing views?

Students should then be provided with a handout summarising the top three negative stereotypes identified by the class as a whole in the pre-class survey. In small groups, students should examine these stereotypes using the discussion prompt below.

> The top three attitudes from the pre-class survey about people experiencing mental illness have been collated and are given in the handout. Do you think these stereotypes are representative of a person experiencing mental illness? Why or why not?

Following the small group discussion, an exploratory activity could be facilitated, encouraging students to investigate how negative stereotypes are developed and how these have a profound impact on those experiencing mental illness. After this discussion, a brainstorming or mind-mapping session about the nature of mental illness could also be conducted using the following prompt. This can be conducted in small or large groups, depending on the class environment.

> In the episode of *Star Trek: Voyager* we watched today, Lieutenant Tuvok is portrayed as a logical and controlled person, able to distance himself from his emotions. In contrast, Ensign Suder is shown to be a person with violent tendencies. After the mind-meld, however, the characteristics of these two protagonists switch: Lieutenant Tuvok becomes violent, while Ensign Suder gains control over his emotions. In what ways can this switch be considered representative of mental illness?

Finally, it is recommended that students complete a reflective study, either in class or as a take-home task. An example of such a reflective study is provided below. This self-discovery activity is designed to allow students to develop an understanding of the threshold concept of realising the person with the mental illness is primarily a person. Given that this task is likely to be very personal and challenging for some students, it is recommended that these reflections are kept private. At the end of the class (or at the start of the next class if the activity is done at home), the teacher could facilitate a session about the theory of person-centred practice. This will allow students to relate their personal reflections to clinical practice theory, encouraging deeper contextualised learning.

In the *Star Trek: Voyager* episode we watched today, Captain Janeway acts as a care-giver for her friend and crew member, Lieutenant Tuvok. She encourages him to take care of himself when he starts experiencing symptoms, she convinces him to go to Sickbay to seek medical treatment when he loses control of his emotions, and she supports him through his treatment and recovery. However, during his illness Lieutenant Tuvok often presents with violent tendencies, acting in a disrespectful and insulting manner towards her.

1. Considering Lieutenant Tuvok's behaviour, how was Captain Janeway able to give him the support he needed without negatively stereotyping him?
2. What strategies can mental health practitioners put into place to treat people who present with behaviours that conflict with societal norms (such as violent tendencies)?
3. In a mental health setting, do you think you will be able to treat patients experiencing mental illness without letting personal biases or stereotypes influence your decision-making? What factors contribute to your answer?

## SUICIDE

The *Star Trek: Voyager* episode 'Death Wish'[19] presents a confronting interpretation of suicide, providing an opportunity for teachers to highlight the conflict between respect for a person's autonomy and the professional duty of non-maleficence. In the episode, Quinn (a member of an immortal alien race known as the Q Continuum) advocates for self-termination, while another member of his race argues that Quinn is mentally unstable. Quinn does not appear to display signs of mental illness and argues that his life has become futile and meaningless, which should be considered as unendurable suffering. Captain Janeway is left to decide whether to allow Quinn to commit suicide or whether to return Quinn to the Q Continuum, where he will be imprisoned for eternity.

While the episode is at times humorous, the over-arching themes covered in 'Death Wish' are complex and likely quite challenging for students, particularly since Quinn ultimately takes his own life.[19]

Attitudes and beliefs about death, and in particular suicide, are often deeply ingrained in culture and religion, so the teacher will have to be aware that this episode could prompt strong responses from students. We therefore suggest that this episode should be watched individually by students prior to attending class. Additionally, students should be provided with a content warning, highlighting that the episode contains a portrayal of suicide.

## STAR TREK: VOYAGER: 'DEATH WISH'[19]

At the beginning of the episode, the Voyager crew are investigating what they think is an unusual comet, and an attempt is made to teleport part of the comet aboard for further study. However, instead of a piece of a comet, a man identifying himself as Quinn appears. The Captain discovers that Quinn has been held captive inside the comet for 300 years. During these discussions Quinn notices Kes, who is a member of a race known as the Ocampa, with a lifespan of approximately nine years.[26] In a matter-of-fact tone, Quinn notes that he envies Kes's short life expectancy, because his own strongest desire is to die.

Quinn then proceeds to make a grand speech where he experiments with different last words. At its conclusion he gestures in the air to use his Q powers, but rather than Quinn disappearing as he apparently intended, all the male crew members on Voyager disappear instead. As the Captain and the remainder of her crew try to determine how to get their fellow crew members back, another member of the Q Continuum appears. Q is a recurring character in many episodes of *Star Trek: The Next Generation, Star Trek: Deep Space Nine* and *Star Trek: Voyager.* Regular audiences of *Star Trek* will be familiar with Q, as his appearances typically cause chaos for the Starfleet crew.[27] In this instance, Q's mission is to return Quinn to his confinement. Q returns the missing crew members to the ship, and is about to send Quinn back to the comet. Before Q is able to complete this task, however, Quinn requests asylum from Captain Janeway, but before the Captain can make a decision, a game of hide-and-seek ensues between Quinn and Q. Quinn continually transports the ship and its crew to places outside normal space and time, with Q quickly finding them. This game becomes increasingly dangerous, threatening to destroy the ship. Captain Janeway proposes a hearing to decide on the matter, in order to ensure the safety of her ship and crew. Q summarises the case as being a dilemma, with the Captain needing to decide Quinn's fate: eternal imprisonment or assisted suicide.

Quinn requests that Lieutenant Tuvok represent him as counsel at the hearing, based on Vulcans' quantified acceptance of ritual suicide for aged Vulcans with life-limiting infirmity. As the hearing begins, Quinn tells the Captain that he wishes to die because he considers immortality to be causing unbearable suffering. Q counters that Quinn is mentally unbalanced, specifically because of this desire for suicide. Lieutenant Tuvok, however, argues that desire for suicide alone cannot be considered as proof of mental instability, pointing out that many cultures consider suicide acceptable in specific circumstances.

Q's argument turns to highlighting the impact that Quinn's suicide, if allowed, would have on the Continuum, changing the fundamental nature of their immortal society. This seems like a strong point until Lieutenant Tuvok reminds those present that the Q Continuum has previously executed members of the Continuum without damaging the society as a whole.

Q's final argument contends that Quinn's life has had value not just for the Continuum but also for other races, in this case humans. He brings three representatives to the ship: Sir Isaac Newton, Maury Ginsberg (an engineer from the 1960s) and Commander William Riker (a Starfleet officer and First Officer of the USS Enterprise in *Star Trek: The Next Generation*).[28] Q shows that Quinn was responsible for Sir Isaac Newton's discovery of gravity, as well as helping Maury Ginsberg save the Woodstock concert after the sound system was damaged, and for saving the life of Commander Riker's ancestor.

The hearing then turns to focus on Quinn's side of the argument. Lieutenant Tuvok shows Captain Janeway the area where Quinn has been imprisoned for centuries. Since Quinn will be returned to confinement in the comet if the Captain does not grant him asylum, Lieutenant Tuvok suggests that Quinn's quality of life should be a consideration. This is followed by a discussion about cultural attitudes concerning suicide. Captain Janeway raises the double-effect principle, considering the ethical justification of an action that primarily seeks to reduce suffering, even if the same action could ultimately result in, or hasten, death. In order for this principle to apply, Lieutenant Tuvok and Quinn need to convince the Captain that living should be considered as suffering in Quinn's case. Quinn decides to show her what his life in the Q Continuum was like, through an analogy she and Lieutenant Tuvok can understand. Quinn transports the entire hearing to a house in the desert.

The house has an old-world feel to it, with a few other beings sitting silently and disinterestedly outside. Next to the house is a road that seems to have no end. Quinn explains that the road is indeed an endless circuit through the Universe. He explains how he has explored the house, and road, many times, even taking on the roles of other beings and inanimate objects in the scene.

Captain Janeway notes that this does not seem to constitute suffering, so Quinn explains that life was once full of discussion and discovery, but over time everything new has been said or done or experienced, and now there is nothing left to think about or discuss that has not been considered many times before.

In the ageing publication being held by one of those at the house, Quinn shows Captain Janeway an article he wrote about his wish to die, an article that led to the Q press being shut down. Quinn explains how he kept speaking out, and how that ultimately resulted in his imprisonment. Q argues that Quinn was confined for his own good, to protect him from self-harm. Quinn has a different perspective: that his opinions on the right of an individual to self-termination posed a threat to the collective Q society, and it was for that reason that he had been imprisoned in the comet for centuries.

Quinn concludes his argument for asylum by claiming that he has nothing left to do or live for, and that continued existence would be unendurable. He challenges the Captain, who is known for her curiosity, to consider what her own life would be like if there were no questions left to ask. He concludes by explaining that, while others might consider immortality desirable, for those living with it, eternal life ultimately becomes more like an unwanted, unendurable disease.

Captain Janeway eventually decides in Quinn's favour, granting him asylum aboard Voyager. Her judgement notes that ultimately the choice for what to do with his life rests with Quinn, but she still feels responsible for any role she plays in facilitating that choice, if it ends in his suicide.

Captain Janeway adjourns the hearing, encouraging Quinn to carefully explore the new experience of being mortal before deciding whether or not to end his life. A little later, as she is contemplating possible roles for Quinn on the ship, the Captain is summoned by the Doctor where she learns that Quinn is dying, having taken a rare poison with no known cure.

## LEARNING ACTIVITIES

Learning activities associated with the episode 'Death Wish' should allow students to expand their understanding about autonomy and non-maleficence in the context of the threshold concept of person-centred practice.[19] Successful person-centred practice necessitates that practitioners are able to examine the strengths and weakness of their own views, as well as understand someone else's perspective, even when that perspective is fundamentally different, or even in opposition to, their own. In particular, students should be encouraged to look beyond a patient's behaviour to consider the person's lived experience.

At the start of the class, students should consider the following discussion prompt in small groups. This is designed to contextualise the issues raised in 'Death Wish' into contemporary society.

> In the episode 'Death Wish,' Quinn wants to commit suicide, ending a life he considers to be unendurable. In present-day society, there are several advocates for assisted suicide in cases of terminal diseases. There are also many who oppose this idea. Why do you think this concept is so controversial?

Another activity that could be used is a more focused discussion based on one of the questions below. These questions are likely to be quite challenging for students, as they consider ideas that may conflict with their personal or traditional knowledge. We therefore recommend that this question should be considered in small groups, allowing students the opportunity for shared learning as they discuss their opinions.

> - Q states that his society needs to control those who interfere with its smooth function. Is mental illness considered a disruption to our society? Why or why not?
> - Quinn claims that the other members of the Q Continuum locked him away for their safety, not his own, because they feared him. How could this be considered true for our society's current mental health treatment strategies?

- Q says that there would be chaos if individuals could choose between life and death. Do you, as a group, agree? Why or why not?
- Do you think a patient who advocates for euthanasia or assisted suicide because of their terminal illness should be considered as experiencing a mental illness? Why or why not? What about if the person's illness is not terminal?

In order to allow students to explore their own views as well as those of others more deeply, we suggest a role-play or mock-debate activity. The role play or mock debate should focus on encouraging students to take on opposing perspectives, as this can help them to understand the situation from diverse perspectives. It is important to note that some roles might be particularly challenging for individual students, depending on their own personal life experiences. A suggested list of different perspectives is presented below:

- A person with a terminal illness who advocates for self-termination;
- A doctor who has to adhere to the ethical principles of respect for autonomy, non-maleficence and beneficence;
- The carer of a person with a terminal illness who witnesses the suffering of their loved one;
- A palliative care practitioner who works to facilitate a smooth palliative care journey for those with life-limiting illnesses;
- A person who argues for the sanctity of life;
- A person who advocates for the rights of individuals to choose their manner of death; and
- A judge who must interpret and apply the country's laws.

The final part of the class should allow students to discuss ideas for an assessed task focussing on person-centred practice in the context of medical ethics. An ideal task would be one that provides students the opportunity to choose their research topic (either freely or from a list of suggestions), within the overarching themes of person-centred practice and medical ethics. Allowing students to choose what to explore and how to present their findings can empower them to challenge their own thinking. This assessment task can be designed as a capstone activity, culminating in the sharing of the students' final products of learning at a mini-conference or on the learning management system at the end of the semester. This will encourage shared learning and allow students to consider topics from several different perspectives.

## CONCLUSION

This chapter described the use of two episodes of *Star Trek: Voyager* as a narrative teaching strategy to explore two threshold concepts that contribute to ethical person-centred practice in mental healthcare provision: recognising personal and societal biases leading to fear and stigma associated with mental illness and realising that a person living with a mental illness is primarily a person. Since many episodes of *Star Trek* focus on mental health and well-being, this strategy can also be used to examine other threshold concepts associated with mental illness. Additionally, the *Star Trek* universe addresses many ethical and moral dilemmas in areas such as medical science, science and technology, humanities and social sciences, computer science, law, religious studies and economics. We therefore suggest that *Star Trek* can be an effective narrative teaching strategy to engage students and examine complex ethical and moral concepts in an environment partially removed from traditional biases.

## NOTES

1. C.J.L. Murray, T. Vos, R. Lozano, M. Naghavi, A.D. Flaxman, C. Michaud et al., 'Disability-Adjusted Life Years (DALYs) for 291 Diseases and Injuries in 21 Regions, 1990–2010: A Systematic Analysis for the Global Burden of Disease Study 2010,' *The Lancet* 380, no. 9859 (2012): 2197–223.
2. Australian Institute of Health and Welfare, 'Mental Health Services in Brief 2014,' (Canberra: Australian Institute of Health and Welfare, 2014).
3. C. Lauber, C. Nordt, C. Braunschweig and W. Rossler, 'Do Mental Health Professionals Stigmatize Their Patients?' *Acta Psychiatrica Scandinavica* 113, no. 429 (2006): 51–9.
4. P. Pietikäinen, *Madness: A History* (Oxford: Routledge, 2015).
5. D.R. Edney, 'Mass Media and Mental Illness: A Literature Review' (Ontario: Canadian Mental Health Association, 2004).
6. G. Schomerus, C. Schwahn, A. Holzinger, P.W. Corrigan, H.J. Grabe, M.G. Carta et al., 'Evolution of Public Attitudes About Mental Illness: A Systematic Review and Meta-Analysis,' *Acta Psychiatrica Scandinavica* 125, no. 6 (2012): 440–52.

7. P.W. Corrigan, S.B. Morris, P.J. Michaels, J.D. Rafacz and N. Rüsch, 'Challenging the Public Stigma of Mental Illness: A Meta-Analysis of Outcome Studies,' *Psychiatric Services* 63, no. 10 (2012): 963–73.

8. B.D. Smedley, A.Y. Stith and A.R. Nelson, eds., *Unequal Treatment: Confronting Racial and Ethnic Disparities in Health Care* (Washington, DC: National Academies Press, 2003).

9. J. Groopman, *How Doctors Think* (New York, NY: Mariner Books, 2008).

10. J.H.F. Meyer and R. Land, *Overcoming Barriers to Student Understanding: Threshold Concepts and Troublesome Knowledge* (Oxford: Routledge, 2006).

11. J.H.F. Meyer, R. Land and C. Baillie, *Threshold Concepts and Transformational Learning* (Rotterdam: Sense Publishers, 2010).

12. D. Perkins, 'Constructivism and Troublesome Knowledge,' in *Overcoming Barriers to Student Understanding: Threshold Concepts and Troublesome Knowledge*, ed. J.H.F. Meyer and R. Land (Oxford: Routledge, 2006), 3–19.

13. B. Tanner, 'Threshold Concepts in Practice Education: Perceptions of Practice Educators,' *British Journal of Occupational Therapy* 74, no. 9 (2011): 427–34.

14. J.J. Hughes and J.D. Lantos, 'Medical Ethics through the Star Trek Lens,' *Literature and Medicine* 20, no. 1 (2001): 26–38.

15. L. Pretorius and A. Ford, 'The Needs of the Many Outweigh the Needs of the Few: Teaching Medical Ethics Using Star Trek,' 2017 [previous chapter].

16. C. Chalmers, 'Ethics,' *Star Trek: The Next Generation*, Season 5, Episode 16, screened 29 February 1992 (United States of America: Paramount Pictures, 1992).

17. J. Summers, 'Theory of Healthcare Ethics,' in *Health Care Ethics: Critical Issues for the 21st Century*, ed. E.E. Morrison and B. Furlong (Burlington, MA: Jones & Bartlett Learning, 2014): 3–45.

18. C. Bole, 'Meld,' *Star Trek: Voyager*, Season 2, Episode 16, screened 5 February 1996 (United States of America: United Paramount Network, 1996).

19. J.L. Conway, 'Death Wish,' *Star Trek: Voyager*, Season 2, Episode 18, screened 19 February 1996 (United States of America: United Paramount Network, 1996).

20. 'Star Trek: Voyager,' *Star Trek Database*. Accessed 28 June 2016. Available at: http://www.startrek.com/page/star-trek-voyager.

21. 'Q Aliens,' *Star Trek Database*. Accessed 28 June 2016. Available at: http://www.startrek.com/database_article/q-aliens.

22. 'Vulcans,' *Star Trek Database*. Accessed 28 June 2016. Available at: http://www.startrek.com/database_article/vulcans.

23. 'Betazoids,' *Star Trek Database*. Accessed 28 June 2016. Available at: http://www.startrek.com/database_article/betazoids.
24. 'Mind-Meld, Vulcan,' *Star Trek Database*. Accessed 28 June 2016. Available at: http://www.startrek.com/database_article/mind-meld-vulcan.
25. 'Holodeck,' *Star Trek Database*. Accessed 28 June 2016. Available at: http://www.startrek.com/database_article/holodeck.
26. 'Ocampa,' *Star Trek Database*. Accessed 28 June 2016. Available at: http://www.startrek.com/database_article/ocampa1.
27. 'Q,' *Star Trek Database*. Accessed 28 June 2016. Available at: http://www.startrek.com/database_article/q.
28. 'Riker, William,' *Star Trek Database*. Accessed 28 June 2016. Available at: http://www.startrek.com/database_article/riker-william.

**Acknowledgements** *Star Trek* is a trade mark of CBS Studios Inc.

## BIBLIOGRAPHY

Australian Institute of Health and Welfare. 'Mental Health Services in Brief 2014.' Canberra: Australian Institute of Health and Welfare, 2014.

Bole, C. 'Meld,' *Star Trek: Voyager*, season 2, episode 16, screened 5 February 1996. United States of America: United Paramount Network, 1996.

Chalmers, C. 'Ethics,' *Star Trek: The Next Generation*, season 5, episode 16, screened 29 February 1992. United States of America: Paramount Pictures, 1992.

Conway, J.L. 'Death Wish,' *Star Trek: Voyager*, Season 2, Episode 18, screened 19 February 1996. United States of America: United Paramount Network, 1996.

Corrigan, P.W., S.B. Morris, P.J. Michaels, J.D. Rafacz and N. Rüsch. 'Challenging the Public Stigma of Mental Illness: A Meta-Analysis of Outcome Studies.' *Psychiatric Services* 63, no. 10 (2012): 963–73.

Edney, D.R. 'Mass Media and Mental Illness: A Literature Review.' Ontario: Canadian Mental Health Association, 2004.

Groopman, J. *How Doctors Think*. New York: Mariner Books, 2008.

Hughes, J.J. and J.D. Lantos. 'Medical Ethics through the Star Trek Lens.' *Literature and Medicine* 20 no. 1 (2001): 26–38.

Lauber, C., C. Nordt, C. Braunschweig and W. Rossler. 'Do Mental Health Professionals Stigmatize Their Patients?' *Acta Psychiatrica Scandinavica* 113, no. 429 (2006): 51–9.

Meyer, J.H.F. and R. Land. *Overcoming Barriers to Student Understanding: Threshold Concepts and Troublesome Knowledge*. Oxford: Routledge, 2006.

Meyer, J.H.F., R. Land and C. Baillie. *Threshold Concepts and Transformational Learning.* Rotterdam: Sense Publishers, 2010.

Morrison, E.E. and B. Furlong, eds. *Health Care Ethics: Critical Issues for the 21st Century.* Burlington, MA: Jones & Bartlett Learning, 2014.

Murray, C.J.L., T. Vos, R. Lozano, M. Naghavi, A.D. Flaxman, C. Michaud et al. 'Disability-Adjusted Life Years (DALYs) for 291 Diseases and Injuries in 21 Regions, 1990–2010: A Systematic Analysis for the Global Burden of Disease Study 2010.' *The Lancet* 380, no. 9859 (2012): 2197–223.

Pietikäinen, P. *Madness: A History.* Oxford: Routledge, 2015.

Schomerus, G., C. Schwahn, A. Holzinger, P.W. Corrigan, H.J. Grabe, M.G. Carta et al. 'Evolution of Public Attitudes About Mental Illness: A Systematic Review and Meta-Analysis.' *Acta Psychiatrica Scandinavica* 125, no. 6 (2012): 440–52.

Smedley, B.D., A.Y. Stith and A.R. Nelson, eds. *Unequal Treatment: Confronting Racial and Ethnic Disparities in Health Care.* Washington, DC: National Academies Press, 2003.

*Star Trek Database.* Accessed 28 June 2016. Available at: http://www.startrek.com/database.

Tanner, B. 'Threshold Concepts in Practice Education: Perceptions of Practice Educators.' *British Journal of Occupational Therapy* 74, no. 9 (2011): 427–34.

# INDEX

**A**
Advocacy, 5
*All Saints*, 104, 110
American Medical Association, 8, 46,
    145
Autonomy, 26, 135, 152, 158, 162,
    163

**B**
*Ben Casey*, 40, 46
*Body of Proof*, 40
*Bones*, 40

**C**
Cancer, 5, 12, 14, 24, 42, 136
Cancer prevention, 73, 75, 84
CDC, 9, 46, 59, 62
Celebrity, 5, 6, 72, 74–76, 79, 81, 83,
    84, 118, 125
Celebrity doctor, 72, 75–77, 81, 82,
    84, 85
*Chicago Hope*, 8, 40, 46, 49
Christina Yang, 108

*City Hospital*, 1, 46, 51
Clinical setting, 4, 106
*Combat Hospital*, 40
Confidentiality, 106
Consent, 106, 107, 136
CPR, 8, 10, 17–22, 24–28, 30, 32,
    42–44, 111, 113
Creutzfeldt Jakob disease, 63
CSI, 10, 39–42, 47, 48
Curriculum, 2, 3, 7, 10, 117, 125,
    126

**D**
*28 Days Later*, 61, 66
Decision-making, 101, 116, 158
*Dexter*, 40
Doctor-patient, 1, 3, 107, 134, 152
Doctor-patient relationships, 107
*Doogie Howser, M.D.*, 40
Dr. House, 43, 45, 108
Dr. John Carter, 49
Dr. Mark Greene, 47
Dr. Oz, 47, 48, 74, 77, 90
Dumb Ways to Die, 6, 118, 125

© The Editor(s) (if applicable) and The Author(s) 2017          169
E. Kendal and B. Diug (eds.), *Teaching Medicine and Medical Ethics
Using Popular Culture*, Palgrave Studies in Science and Popular Culture,
DOI 10.1007/978-3-319-65451-5

**E**
Ebola, 57, 62
Educational intervention, 4
*Embarrassing Bodies*, 103
Emergency medicine, 7, 8, 45, 49, 60
ER, 4, 6–8, 10, 12–14, 20, 28, 31, 37, 39–51, 100, 103, 110
Ethics, 1, 3, 7, 11, 17, 133–136, 139, 141, 143, 144, 151, 152, 163

**F**
Facebook, 115, 120, 122, 124, 126–128

**G**
Generation Y, 116
*Grey's Anatomy*, 4, 8, 11, 12, 14, 15, 20, 25, 32, 39, 40, 42, 43, 45–48, 100, 103, 105, 106, 108, 110

**H**
Haemophilia, 136
*Hart of Dixie*, 103
Health campaigns, 5, 117
Health information, 1, 4, 5, 8, 37, 38, 43, 47, 112, 116, 117
HeLa cells, 136, 140
Henrietta Lacks, 136, 140, 145
*Heroes*, 17, 28
HIV, 4, 9, 43, 45, 47, 58, 65
*24 Hours in Emergency*, 103, 107
*House, M.D.*, 19, 31, 40, 41, 43, 45, 103, 105–107, 110

**I**
Infection prevention and control, 10, 56–58, 60–63

Influenza, 59, 136
Instagram, 120, 128

**K**
Kaiser Family Foundation, 4, 8, 11, 15, 45
*King's Cross ER*, 103

**L**
*Law & Order*, 40
LinkedIn, 121, 129

**M**
*M*A*S*H*, 40, 46, 103, 110
Mass media, 1, 2, 6, 41, 50
*Medic*, 20, 23, 25, 26, 32
Medicalisation, 26
Mental health, 11, 150–152, 158, 162, 164
Mental illness, 149–153, 156–158, 162, 164
Meredith Grey, 108
MERs, 57
Millennials, 117
*Monday Mornings*, 40

**N**
*NCIS*, 40
Neoliberal, 38, 39
NIH, 46
*Nip/Tuck*, 40, 104

**O**
*Offspring*, 104
*One Born Every Minute*, 103

**P**
Parkinson's disease, 136
Patient-centred care, 11
Pew Research Center, 116, 117, 128
Pokemon Go, 121, 129
Policymakers, 101, 109, 111
Polio, 136
Popular culture, 1, 2, 4, 6–10, 43, 55, 57, 99–101, 109, 111, 112
Preparedness, 60, 62
*Princess Bride, The*, 60
*Private Practice*, 40, 103, 110
Professionalism, 7, 119, 125–127
Public health, 43, 48, 60, 102, 116–119, 122, 125, 129

**R**
*R.P.A.*, 103, 107
*Rescue 911*, 8, 46
*Resident Evil*, 57, 63

**S**
SARS, 57, 59, 62
*Scrubs*, 3, 12, 15, 40, 100, 103, 105–107, 110
*Shaun of the Dead*, 58, 61, 66
Snapchat, 121, 122, 124, 129
Social media, 5, 6, 10, 115–117, 119–123, 125, 126
*Spiderman*, 63
Spock, 135
Spokesperson, 72–76, 78–84
*St. Elsewhere*, 40, 46

*Star Trek*, 11, 56, 134–138, 140, 141, 144–146, 152, 153, 156–160, 164–167
Storytelling, 42, 152
SunSmart, 77, 78, 91, 92
Symptoms, 4, 153, 158

**T**
*Trapper John, M.D.*, 40
Turk, 108
Twitter, 6, 58, 115–117, 119, 121–130

**V**
Vampires, 63

**W**
WHO, 56
*World War Z*, 61

**X**
*X-Files*, 63

**Y**
YouTube, 61, 121, 129

**Z**
Zombie, 10, 58–64